RUPTURED HEART ....

A CARETAKER'S JOURNEY

By
Suzanne, RN

Vista publishing, Inc.

Edited by Carolyn S. Zagury, MS, RN, CPC

Cover Design by Thomas Taylor of Thomcatt Graphics

Vista Publishing, Inc.
473 Broadway
Long Branch, NJ 07740
(908) 229-6500

Printed and bound in the United States of America

First Edition

ISBN: 1-880254-21-2

Library of Congress Catalog Card Number: 94-61760

U.S.A. Price	$10.95
Canada Price:	$16.95

DEDICATION

To my parents, to my sister and brother

and ...

most of all to my SISTERS.

MEET THE AUTHOR

With an extensive background in publishing, Suzanne has had essays published in the ***L.A. Times***, ***Nurseweek***, a California Nursing publication, in ***The R.N. Times***, and in ***Revolution: The Journal of Nurse Empowerment***. Suzanne also published a journal of arts and letters in Santa Monica, California, for one year.

Suzanne raised her two sons as a single parent and is proud of each of their accomplishments. She currently gives lectures to doctors and nurses on the issue of domestic violence. She also works as a consultant for a major insurance company. Suzanne describes herself as an artist in search of truth, beauty, and holiness.

A strong love of the nursing profession and for the patients for whom she has cared, were the basis of her willingness to share the troubled and often heart breaking experiences Suzanne dealt with during her nursing career. She hopes that by sharing even her most personal thoughts and feelings that nurses will gain the strength to realize their self-esteem and to insist on the honor that belongs to nurses in every field of our profession.

AUTHOR'S NOTES

While referring to nurses in the feminine, I wish to make clear my support of male nurses as well. Nevertheless, since the majority of us are female, it is to the women nurses that much of this is directed, since male nurses (in my experience) have not had the same "assertiveness" issues and have not been as "discounted" as female nurses. If this is a misconception on my part, my apologies and empathy go out to you.

THANK YOU TO:

Len, PhD, for helping me to know what I will and will not do. Your voice goes with me;

Scott, champion of my words;

Dick-the-Doctor, for keeping the memories of childhood;

Dana, LCSW, for inspiring the art of holding people accountable;

E. B. Spiller, MD, for saving my life;

Lana-lips, my birthday soulmate, for your support;

Holly, for nurturing my words. "Words are movement from within." - I Ching;

Margaret, Marlene, and Barbara, kindred spirits;

Norman, and his can-do example;

Ed, for helping me to keep the faith, reminding me, "It will get better!" Godspeed;

Dave and Abbo, for lovingly supporting my work;

Jan, my sponsor, for her willingness to become a steady friend despite days of "unwanted, unloved, and alone";

Dorothy and David, for their enduring support;

Carole, for trusting me, and inspiring my trust;

Anita, sister-of-the-soul: the "curse" can be banished!

Larry, for making me laugh;

Alicia-Snow-White, for all you are;

S. K. and J. T., my sons, whose gift of presence has nourished me, challenged me to reach for Grace, given me strength to continue, and rewarded me beyond all words;

Tim, once my husband, and Sean, once my lover, whose significance moved me towards transformation;

Barbara and Fran, nurses of the highest order, for their inspiration;

Carolyn, for supporting me when an earthquake upset the deadline;

Alanon and the 12 Steps of Alcoholics Anonymous and my Higher Power, without which these pages might have been blank;

All souls past, present, and future, who have been woven into the fabric of my life;

ALL OF MY DAYS, MY LIFE, THAT GREAT MYSTERIOUS GIFT WHICH TELLS ME WHAT IT WANTS OF ME.

Suzanne, 1994

TABLE OF CONTENTS

TABLE OF CONTENTS

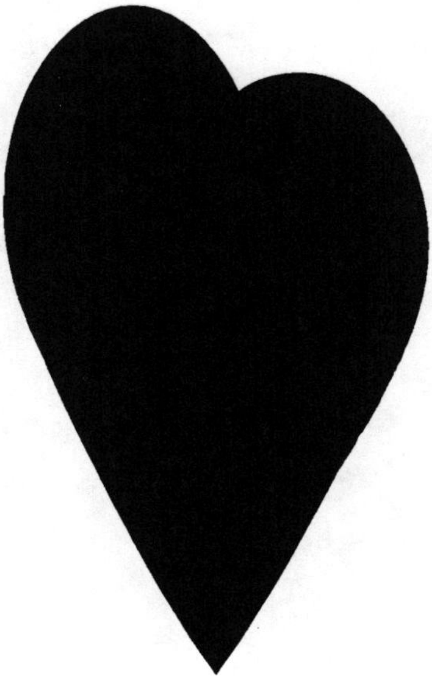

"Medicine
must always
be accompanied
by prayer and
good thoughts."

Medicine Man to a Follower

From ***Book of the Hopi*** by Frank Waters
Penguin Books. 1972.

PREFACE

I don't know how many people I've put my hands on - don't know how many people I've touched. Literally or figuratively, but my experiences during fifteen years of nursing have prompted me to write these words. They are privileged words, for few in life have the opportunity to see humans at their most poignant moments.

These are also words of revolution. What other term can be used to describe the dramatic effects of the past decade upon our changing health care system? The very personal stories which appear are about a rupture - the heart of a healer, in the art of "healing," and in tolerance for the startling affects caused by our changing population, technology, and reimbursement practices. Heaven, or Providence, help us. Florence, Clara - your archetypal sisters, nursing muses - are you listening? If you have any influence, through the ethers, from the ages, inspire us - don't let us down now!

Suzanne, RN

ONE

ECHOES, PREVIEWS

Large, imposing, gothic. This hundred year-old fortress intimidates, looms. Learning Hospital.

I am assigned to work on the 7th floor. Each floor above and below is identical in floor plan. Each is reached either by a slow and gasping elevator, or by a heart-taxing stairwell. I've chosen the latter. Out of breath, I pause, look around. All seems quiet - the kind of unsettling quiet which makes your skin tingle. I walk timidly through the silent hallway. Various stations are abandoned as per the latest "cutbacks" and/or nursing shortages; they bear the resin of sickness, healing, dying. Beyond, like faint dream-voices coming louder now, I hear the demands and cries of the poor and uninsured, spilling into hallways, pulling at hurried nurses whose tread (and re-tread) are worn thin.

I pause before turning the corner; before being swallowed into the noise. Am I ready? I have been given a glimpse of what is to come. This urgency, this sense of doom, is the first sign of what will ten years later afflict the medical system as a whole.

This building is to become a symbol for that "system," as I enter it, work in it, and, finally begin to leave it, never able, fully, to recover from the shock of that first day as a Registered Nurse.

I turn the corner. The sights match the sounds as I see harried nurses, hurrying by with clanging bottles, syringes.

I see sheet-swathed patients, six-to-a-room, in hallways, in niches. I am overwhelmed, but squelch the feeling to turn and run. I have just completed four years of schooling; pre-requisite classes, feverish studies, night classes in chemistry, algebra, developmental psychology, and speech.

A single parent whose husband left and moved away five years before, I have put children in day-care, become the recipient of food stamps and medical relief, in order to make the trek. I have taken numerous clinical tests and answered multiple multiple-choice questions. I'm not going to quit now!

I try to remember what nursing school gave me. I make the mental search, as I will do over and over in the years to come, for EMPATHY ....

EMPATHY *

She lay curved over the bedside table, a pillow supporting her abdomen and chest. A thin, pale, washed-out blonde, she fidgeted nervously, trying to get situated. We jumped. Despite her apparent frailty, she took command. And we students wanted to please her, to soothe.

Her gaping gown revealed a bony spine. She shivered as the doctor deftly painted her with the yellowish tincture. Not a drop or a dribble. Everything was ready.

She grasped me with a spindly hand as I stood in front of her.

"You're so cold!" she exclaimed. Indeed, my hands were like ice. Looking at me and smiling, she wrapped her fingers around mine.

"Are you ready?" the doctor asked gently. Her head motioned in response, the face now submerged in a pillow.

The needle punctured her; I could hear the dull pop as it made its way through her back, near the affected lung.

Posterior insertion: the cold medical terminology clashed with fleshy reality. The doctor retracted the plunger; bloody fluid filled the syringe. She coughed. I winced.

"The pressure is building!" she said, still muffled by the pillow, as though trying to smother the discomfort. I felt myself holding a breath. The doctor continued, methodically, to withdraw the fluid, looking, I thought, like a human mosquito. I immediately countered this thought with a medical cliché: *"He's doing what needs to be done."*

But was he? I wondered what next? More chemo? Surgery? Was this discomfort worth it ... worth what?

Her grip in mine became firmer. It was a sustained, strong grasp. Finally, her raspy voice: "Do you have enough?"

"All through." said the doctor, punctuating the reply with a quick withdrawal of the syringe and a brisk nod to my fellow student, who applied a pressure gauze.

"We'll let you know the results," he said, barely grazing her shoulder as he left. She didn't reply.

* "Empathy," originally published in ***Imprint***, National Student Nurses Association magazine. Reprinted with permission

The specimens were labeled, placed on a stained green towel and carried away, like the cancer which was probably causing the internal bleeding, making her cough, making her pale, making her brave.

Emerging from her pillow, she looked at me, still clutching my hand. Her brown eyes were accepting; though I wanted to cry for her, her dignified gaze precluded it. She seemed serene.

Smiling, she lifted my hands in hers.

"I warmed you!" she said.

At the great medical center, I, a day person, work nights. No choice. New grads pay dues. I fear the loss of my "beauty and intelligence," as I jokingly, but truthfully, tell non-nurse friends. I have constant sleep hunger and obsessive sleep-seeking behavior. Life begins to center on the next nap. With my two young children in school, I'm unable to leave the phone off the hook. My face soon takes on the "moonlight tan" for which the night workers are famous; that waxy blue-toned appearance which stems from being under false light. My fears become silly, my exposure to light would age me doubly fast; I would join the night of the living dead. Single, I'd miss meeting a man while napping, and be too tired for one if I found him! To paraphrase Shakespeare: sleeplessness magnifies all care!

Still, the hospital "night" is fascinating, especially in an institution such as this; personnel, patients, are of a different cloth. A different rhythm flows in the middle of the night. Patients wander halls, wide awake. In the basement, where I occasionally have to go to pick up a supply or two, radios blare, card games are shuffled. The Zombies come out - creatures in far-out clothing who mumble and shuffle and disappear into shadows. They seem to "float" through the stairwells and porticos as wraiths in a lost city. Many years later, in the aftermath of hospital shootings, security will need to be tightened. Many years later, illnesses which we couldn't have imagined will invent themselves and cause a terror of their own.

Now, the task at hand for this graduate nurse is to learn about "Rules and Regulations," and "leadership."

TWO

RULES AND REGULATIONS

I start as a new grad, as an "Interim Permitee," - a limbo category for those whose Board Exam results are pending. The photograph shows me scowling, not smiling, in the wake of the flash and the I.D. number and the pages of dress codes, policies, rules and regulations.

For those who haven't seen one, the following is an incident report. Summaries of "untoward events" - the uncharted background of an incident or event - are described here. These are the summations of incompetence, annoyance, maliciousness, or horror. The report is meant to be an account of internal difficulties which need solutions and prevention. Incident reports explain major and minor irritations - and the day when we don't do one - when we were too busy or the shift took on a life of its own - is the day we wish we had.

INCIDENT REPORT

COMPLETE IMMEDIATELY FOR EVERY INCIDENT AND SEND TO ADMINISTRATOR.

CONFIDENTIAL REPORT OF INCIDENT (**NOT** a part of Medical Record)

PATIENT: John Doe (aka Houdini) **AGE:** 45 **SEX:** M **ROOM:** 777

ADMITTING DIAGNOSIS: Hydrocephalus

ATTENDING PHYSICIAN: Dearth **DATE OF INCIDENCE:** 8/8/88

WERE BED RAILS UP? yes **WAS SAFETY BELT IN USE?** Yes/restrained

WAS PATIENT RATIONAL? No

SEDATIVES? NARCOTICS? DOSES: TIME: NA

TIME DOCTOR WAS CALLED: On Scene

TIME DOCTOR RESPONDED: Immediately

I NOTIFIED DR.: Dearth

BY: Suzanne, RN ___ RN ___ LVN (circle)

NURSES ACCOUNT OF THE INCIDENT: (INCLUDE EXACT LOCATION, etc.) (Use more paper if necessary)

Patient drank own urine.

Incident reports were filed regarding all of the following events and stories.

HOUDINI

"You're beautiful, can I have some water?" asked a middle aged man with aquiline features and aqua eyes.

"Hydrocephalus" was his diagnosis; his mind was clouded with what his attention desired: water. He was a man driven: every glass, every bottle, a potential quenching. He was a danger to himself, and disoriented. To protect him from his disease and from his obsession, his hands and feet were restrained.

I reported this to the day shift. I took his efforts at manipulation in good humor. I reported that. I reported to the oncoming nurses and to the new students.

One student came in late.

While preparing to leave at the end of the shift, I heard groans and laughs from the six-bed ward; the ashen-faced student and I collided as I rushed to see what caused the commotion. I found the patient twisted like a pretzel, hands and arms still tied, drinking from the urinal which the student had left on his bedside table.

"Ahh!" said the man, a convoluted smile on his face. We didn't know whether to be shocked or to laugh. The urinal was removed; Houdini looked at me with a sly face.

I did what nurses always do when "untoward" events occur: I filed an incident report.

THREE

LEADERSHIP

My bewilderment brings me a disadvantage, for I am summed up by the staff as GREEN. They announce that they will not accept all of the patients; that it's only fair for me take a ward of six patients for myself. In charge, but not knowing how to TAKE charge, in a role reversal, I take the assignment that THEY give me, in addition to my "charge" responsibilities start and regulate all intravenous bottles and medications, be accountable for the well being of all the patients (32) on the ward, initiate actions with worsening patients, take and "implement" doctors' orders, report on "incidents," SUPERVISE (?) employees and console them as needed, report all data to the oncoming shift ....

In nursing school, they called this 'reality shock.' There was more to come; we are called to choose, to act in conscience, sometimes with dire consequences.

CORONER'S CASE

Rounds. Room 225: bed 4. Strangely still. No, NOT BREATHING! Pulse, faint. Call a code! As I am about to begin CPR, his stomach contracts, a rumble starts, blood gushes from him, nose, mouth, everywhere. My uniform is soaked as I reach for suction, no time to be horrified.

I turn it on. Nothing, none. NOW I am horrified. Call for another, portable. STAT. The intern comes to intubate, but is thwarted by a crimson tidal wave.

The portable suction is brought; it also malfunctions. We are frustrated and frantic - and helpless. Another suction unit, found in one of the abandoned stations, arrives too late. The man has drowned in his own blood.

The intern is disgusted. I must continue my rounds in a blood-soaked uniform until one of the aides finds me a scrub-suit. I am sick at heart, and we are all unaware of the threat which is to thrust itself in another few years into our lives - the AIDS virus. For now, it has been merely a bloody battle which we lost. He is quickly sent to the morgue, now a coroner's case. Sudden, death.

I file an incident report.

ACCOUNTABLE

We are told that the unconscious man, hit by a car, leg broken, is to be seen by an orthopedic resident. We are told that the resident has not been in, but we are under strict orders not to change the dressing. We are told that the interns need the experience. The man was injured six days ago, with, heretofore, no dressing change.

I decide to take responsibility - and I will be sorry. I approach the comatose man - a transient - and begin to unravel the dressing; the stench of rotted flesh assaults me; I turn my head and gag. I proceed again; the man deserves attention.

I get closer to the sordid flesh, closer to death as I unwind the green-tinged, rotting bandage. As if to warn me, a handful of maggots spill, wriggling and eyeless, from within the decayed wound. My intention is sabotaged; I bolt to the bathroom, retching.

When I return, one of the aides has put a clean towel over the site; the creatures are gone.

We leave a message with the Orthopedic service, we make out an incident report, we inform the supervisor.

The man dies two hours later. Our voices, protesting, echo and fall still amongst the resin of bodies and spirits; his has joined them. The aide says a prayer for him; I see her broad black hands closing his eyes. We say "Amen."

PRINCIPLES

> "As your go through your careers, you will never get into trouble if you remember your basic principles and the ABC's - airway, breathing, circulation - do no harm, maintain the integrity of the patient and, if possible, have the greatest attribute of all, empathy. Put yourself in the patient's shoes - slippers - and you will be, not just a good nurse, you will be the finest nurse."

Nursing Instructor
Pasadena City College

The echo never quite leaves me, the scowl is often on my face when confronting bureaucratic repression. I calculate doses, assess vital signs, evaluate the bodies, minds, and spirits of the sick. The sick need me, the dying need me, the living-dead need me. They need my spirit, my nurturing bent, my gentle compassion. In the face of short-staffing, overcrowding, poor working conditions and lack of supplies, they receive very little of this, the best of me; the rules, the numbers, the crowded hallways pull at me and mock my purpose. Nursing becomes, at worst, a great sieve attempting to strain, now and then, a dose a millimeter, of healing.

In the beginning, I brim with compassion, purpose, empathy. I remember the lecture by my favorite instructor, Mrs. Helbing, who said, "we need good nurses so badly." In the end, I learn that my part in this daily "be-tough/make do" drama is somehow skewed; a childhood framed by my father's alcoholism taught me to bat my head against the wall in attempts to "fix the unfixable," and to accept the unacceptable. I learned an "all or nothing" approach to life, which leaves one feeling helpless.

The hospital system we have today, and the lack of recognition by physicians and the public regarding the contribution of nurses, feeds right into this attitude. It is called "martyrdom," and leads to illness, to burnout, to addiction. Feeling helpless to change things, I often awoke before work praying for a healing attitude, and to come to no harm. The prayer would fail me, in a big way, as I struggled with those demons. But evolution takes time.

Below are examples of the best and the worst of my days as a nurse at the giant institution.

IRONY, PATHOS, HUMOR, APPRECIATION

- An alcoholic, belly swollen, talks to the wall. He thinks he is in Vietnam, and the president is Lyndon Johnson.
- An addict tells me she hates needles.
- A would-be suicide tells me I am easy to talk to.
- An old woman, full of arthritic pain, thanks me for the moment I take to massage her back.
- An alcoholic, lungs full of pus, has two tubes beneath her breasts, draining into large bottles. "I've always got a bottle with me," she laughs.
- I call the supervisor. The L.V.N. who was to work with me is sick. "Just do the best you can," she says.

Tonight I TELL THEM: I won't take a room full of patients. After a brief silence, "We're in this together!" says one of the aides, the one who said "Amen." It is my turn to offer a prayer of thanks.

WOMAN TO WOMAN

If we want to measure the accomplishments of the feminist movement, then we are better not to look within the hospital environment, for the way in which women treat women in this setting is abysmal. No matter what the reasons, nurses continue to give great compassion to everyone but each other. Similarly, women, when making the leap into medicine (or other predominantly male professions), often take on a superior, rather than supportive attitude; a heartless approach, with predictable results.

A friend is coming to town, and I call to ask the nursing office if I can trade with another nurse. "The schedule is made out a month ahead of time," I am told. It is my first realization that this supervisor's main goal is not to have compassion for fellow nurses. It is to have a warm, experienced body on the unit. "Sorry," she says. No, she is not sorry. I understand her dilemma, but there is no room in this system (and it does not change over the years) for appreciation of staff's personal life. No recognition for the hard work I have done. I call in sick.

In this great exciting learning center, I meet several women who are in the process of becoming physicians. I say to myself, "That's great! Maybe now women will have compassionate care instead of the patronizing pat on the head which we often receive from those doctors who dub women's concerns as "hysterical." I am introduced to a resident in internal medicine. I give her a smile, introduce myself as the charge nurse. She turns her head without any acknowledgment whatsoever, as if to say, "So?"

I meet many more women who are studying to be "dear and glorious physicians," and many who have the same bitchy attitude. It's the power game, and I am appalled. They treat nurses as invisible, as if what nurses do is "scut" work. They have turned against their own in the quest for "personal best."

In contrast are the "goddesses," my heroines, who see that we are a team - but don't loose their authority. Yet, I wonder how they keep their sanity in this power-hungry place. I cannot get over it; the way women treat women in the medical profession. And, the result is not contained to physicians versus nurses. The oppression moves down the line: nurses to nurses, nurses to aides, aides to housekeepers, etc.

I admit that I have also reacted to this kind of treatment and been bitchy to someone else in kind. The realization propels me into despair; after all that women have been striving for, "competition" with each other still impedes us all. When women deprecate other women, we are rendered as helpless as if we had never had any voice at all. It makes me angry, and then it makes me very sad.

THE LAST STRAW

Eleven p.m. As I begin tonight, I am in the step-down unit, "semi-critical" (hah!) patients. The pay-back comes: the other RN is ill. An L.V.N. is coming "later." She is excluded from IV monitoring. Six patients, sick, sick, sick patients. During the course of the night:

One patient stops breathing and dies despite prolonged resuscitation efforts. One is comatose. One deteriorates, needing frequent blood assessment. One bleeds, requiring transfusion. All have IV medications due at staggered times. The intern is new and needs to be advised. As a patient is going into respiratory arrest, the fledgling doctor says, "I think I'll get a blood gas." I hand him the ambu bag, holler for help, and tell him, "No doctor, we need to start CPR." The shift is a disaster, with no end!

As the supervisor is called to ANOTHER floor to assist CPR, a patient is admitted to the outside ward, for which I am responsible. The patient has TB. and the other patient in the room is complaining. Our patient who has coded has expired, and there is no help to do post-mortem care. I cover him with a sheet, close the curtain, and wait for help to arrive - as other "full-moon effects" - for it is a night of a full moon - continue to erupt.

I get through the night but, at the end of the shift, collapse in tears. There have been too many shifts like theses, hardly ever a time to sit down, to regroup. Yet, I feel ashamed. Gone are my childhood visions: soothing a fevered brow, making things right ... Something has gone terribly wrong. I haven't yet learned to accept my limitations. I see them as indications that I am fatally flawed as a being: a failure. I haven't yet learned that before we can obtain respect from others we must first be able to love ourselves. And, if we can't accept limitations in ourselves, we certainly can't tolerate them in others.

My skewed thinking continued: if only I knew what it was, I could fix it ...

FOUR

FIXING IT

Another hospital might be the answer. That will make it better. A smaller, private, "cushy" hospital ...

In intensive care, coronary care, I learn to monitor arterial lines, assist with "Swan-Ganz" insertion - a special intravenous line which monitors the capability of the heart to squeeze it's juice from one chamber to the other and vessels and capillaries of the human body. I fine-tune the art of measuring minute drops of urine, come to recognize euphoria as a sign of low oxygen or hypoxia, - impending doom. I come to know patterns of breathing and skin tones which ring "alarm" signals in a nurses' brain, so that with luck, timing, and calm, she will be able to intervene in these situations.

I study for and earn the certificate of C.C.R.N., a prestigious acknowledgment by critical care nurses which is awarded after much preparation, experience, and focus. The certificate recommended and "congratulated" by hospital supervisors, but not compensated. It costs over $100.00 to take the exam, and we are not reimbursed.

I encounter "super nurse syndrome" - in which nurses are extremely critical of one another, ruthlessly competitive and cut-throat. And, worse, unrelenting in their own self-criticism. Further, I see that greed and the fear of lawsuits sometimes precludes acts of compassion. My witnessing the amputation of the hand of a dying man showed me to what extent this fear prevailed. No, this wouldn't work. What I wanted - to be considered competent and compassionate and effective - could not be found here. Continuing to look on the outside for inner validation, I decided to try emergency.

EMERGENCY, E.R. The "land of ER." Here, I might make myself heard. Here, machines are not what challenges me; here, I can teach and soothe - and, I come to understand later, rescue.

The echo, the diorama continues: shined bland floors, the sound of creosote soles squeaking, gurneys rattling, the smell of disinfectant and metal and body waste. White-on-white uniforms and pajama-clad patients dancing with IV poles, curtains drawn, beds made, and sheets pulled over stilled faces; doctors lecturing or scolding. Supervisors in caps with clipboards reminding, reprimanding, fidgeting, conciliating. Nurses tending, fixing, soothing.

And always, ALWAYS, charts, reports, copies, RECORDS.

I carry with me a "noble" sensibility and a serious demeanor. Both need reshaping - I must learn to toughen up, to be more realistic. Or, perhaps less so. but I have not taken, and no one has written, the Zen of Nursing. So, I get stumped on the moral issues, the dramatic ones, on my own dwindling reserve. I wonder, after five years, if I am burning out. Instead of admitting it, I do what I have always done - I persevere.

I rest, I go from full-time to part time to per diem and back again. I take courses, upgrade my knowledge, recertify in required areas, drop the C.C.R.N. - which requires taking 100 C.E.U.'s (continuing education units) and other requirements, which I as a single parent, have little time to pursue.

I persevere: what keeps me going are patients, the MOMENTS of satisfaction and humor. I am especially touched by the old folks, who inspire me to poetry.

OLD WINNIE

Oh Mother, see what I am become:
These folds of flesh,
Once smooth orbs of pleasure,
Now fall like unclaimed letters.

These legs, one loving vines,
Now teeter, bowed and knotted,
Lest these eyes misjudge
And send all parts of me into
Splintering unconsciousness.

These teeth
Can chatter on their own
While I drool foolishly
Like a babe.

And I wish I could hear you once more,
Telling me to close my legs,
And be a lady,
So I could laugh once more
And run away again
And feel with my fingers
The dimple in his chin.
Is this my pay for living sin?

FREDERICK'S TICKER

I took my med-sin
Take 'bout ten a day.
One fer ever' organ
That's what the doctor say.

He say, you take 'em all
but don't take this one
'cept oncet a day
an' stay out' the sun.

If you feel like palp-ations,
yer ticker talkin'
then you gotta set,
'stead o' walkin'.

He say call me if yer heart's a beatin',
or if yer legs're heavy feelin',
or if yer belly's gettin' puffy,
or yer breathin's gettin huffy.

Leastwise don't you worry none,
these pills'll get the job done,
they'll keep you 'roun' fer years to come.
Ain't it fun?

WE MUST LAUGH

Frantic, the best description of the day. All types of patients, young and old, gnarled and smooth, cultured and uncouth, presented themselves to us, we two nurses and one doctor.

Chest pain, belly pain, psychic pain; monitors, IV's, dipsticks, needlesticks. Bedpans, emesis basins, betadine, iodine, lidocaine - kill the pain.

a woman comes to the window with belly pain. She's chubby, wearing a robe, slippers, curlers. She is young, unmarried.

We give her a cup, say "fill it up," send her to the "bano" for a sample of urine.

The other nurse, the doctor and I move in a rhythm: now here now there. Keep the rhythm flowing, keep it all going.

"Nurse, nurse!" my co-worker goes to answer.

"Suzanne, Suzanne!" I rush to investigate.

"Waah, waah, waah!" I hear - is it what I think I hear?

In the bathroom, a baby is being born. It's head is aiming for the toilet bowl, it's mother's face is one of shock and surprise. My co-worker is supporting her.

"Doctor, Doctor!" I holler, ordering a STAT isolette, a "delivery pack," and sterile scissors.

The doctor, in his preppie shirt and saddle oxfords, moves with lightning speed - literally "catching" the infant before it learns to swim. We wrap the baby and rush it to the vacant bed next to the injured worker. The doctor suctions and examines it, a girl, and puts her into the isolette, turning to the man with the cut fingers whose eyeballs are popping out of his head. The doctor turns to him and says, "all in a day's work!" before returning to the mother to deliver the placenta.

The mother, who did not know she was pregnant, was reunited with her newborn daughter shortly thereafter, once proper infection control precautions were taken.

TODOS

Wanting to build a rapport with the Mexican child who spoke English, I asked, "How do you say 'ouch' in Spanish?"

He pondered this.

"Aye!" he finally answered, giggling.

* * * * * * * * * * *

The dark-haired Latin, dusty from work, showed me his cut finger.

"Allergica contra medicina?" I asked in my "patchwork" Spanish.

"No." He answered.

"Las bacunas contra tetana, todas?"

"Yes, I've had a tetnus shot." he answered in perfect English.

We killed ourselves laughing.

PARAMEDIC

He had a very singular talent: he would stretch a latex glove over the top of his head, just over his nostrils, making it stretch upwards and elongate, distorting his face into a cartoon. Then he would blow through his nose until the glove around his eyes and above his head inflated. He resembled an alien rooster. With each breath he would look more and more stupid, more hilarious. The glove would pull tighter against his nose, stretching it higher, flattening his eyebrows, squishing his eyeballs. We would laugh until we cried!

And always, in this alley of audacity, in this room of rooms, there were reasons to cry.

THE JOGGER

He was too young. I can see his face now and though I never saw his face alive, I can tell you he was too young.

Though his pupils are dilated in death, I see that his eyes are blue and once - a very short time ago - full of life. His body was warm, his muscles firm. They served him well. But, he hadn't bargained for the heart to fail. Perhaps if he had seen a doctor before he started jogging, or told someone about the chest pain ... but no, he was young and fit. It would go away.

It didn't go away; it overpowered him in a wave of disbelief and even as he was drowning in his pain, he kept thinking no, this isn't happening. It showed in his face the way last thoughts often do, "I was only jogging, what is happening here?"

I see his face and I wish I could answer the question but what-ifs and whys are never answered, and I see that my feelings are showing and I worry about that. I know that I'll awaken tonight and see his face. I wonder how long I'll continue to see these faces and still be a calm presence wearing white. How long I will be a nurse? What if I did something else for a living? Why do these faces haunt me?

They are the faces of mortality. Life and death are incompatible, in the same instant. This instant, this forever moment, cooling warm and stagnant sigh, appeals to my belief, beckons to hope, even in the abandoning.

No faith, no philosophy has truly prepared me. Like him, I am caught by surprise. It will not go away.

Life is precious.

MORE RULES AND REGULATIONS
OR:
I DIDN'T GO TO NURSING SCHOOL FOR THIS

Some aggravations make a nurse wince and act as a thorn in one's side, like this note from the supervisor.

Suzanne:

Fill out this form for our reimbursement - January
Request for Attendance at Outside Education Program.

1. Submit this request through your immediate supervisor so that he/she may offer comments to the Director of Nursing.
2. Submit a copy of the program with this request.
3. You will be expected to offer proof of attendance.
4. ALL PROGRAM ATTENDANCE MUST HAVE PRIOR APPROVAL IF REIMBURSEMENT IS EXPECTED!

Supervisor Comments: ______________________________

____

____

____

____

____

Signature: ______________________ Date: ______________

Supervisor Signature: _________________________________

Date: ________ Approved: Yes: _____ No: _____

LIST OF TERMS

On a good day in E.R., humor, albeit dark, prevails. It helps to alleviate our pain, as well as yours. Here's a list I created, one slow, listless day. One on which one dares not use the "Q" word, (q-u-i-e-t), lest all hell break loose:

STAT = immediately, if not sooner
ETOH = ethyl alcohol
HBD = has been drinking; used in conjunction with ETOH
HYS = hysterical
SOB = short of breath
BIB = brought in by
GRAVIDA = how many times pregnant
PARA = how many times delivered of live infant
MISSED OR INEVITABLE ABORTION = miscarriage
TAB = therapeutic abortion, ie. "abortion" as know by the populace
CYA = cover your ass
AMA = American medical advice
SYNDROME = a bundle of complaints which has no emergent medical explanation
ETIOL = etiology, or cause. Often accompanies syndrome: ETIOL unknown
ACUTE = immediate cause for hospitalization or surgical intervention
CHRONIC = long term syndrome (let the private MD handle it.)
BURNOUT = inability to continue to perform at optimum level due to stress of the job.
TUBE = to intubate, to assist breathing
CODE = cardiac and/or respiratory arrest
DIPSTICK = chemical sticks which, when dipped in body fluid, indicate (by color change) the presence of protein, blood, ketones (abnormal in a diabetic) and other substances
Q-WORD = Euphemism for "quiet." Whatever you do, never, EVER, say this word out loud, unless you want a disaster ...

It was one of those mornings. A visiting doctor strolled through, took a look around. "My it's quiet!" he said. "Now you've done it," I said. And all hell DID break loose.

NURSES' ACCOUNT OF AN INCIDENT

Patient apparently brought in by police for possible drug manufacturing. Smelled of ether; complained of head injuries. Bleeding from left temple; requiring stitches. Vital signs stable, seen by doctor. Sutured by doctor. Neuro-vitals stable, denies loss of consciousness from blow. Patient states, "They beat the shit out of me!" X-rays negative per doctor.

Suddenly, the patient leapt from the gurney and started screaming. This nurse and co-worker scratched in scramble. Profanity by patient, officers. This nurse saw to the safety of other patients by closing doors to rooms, but unable to do so before mace used by officers in their effort to subdue patient.

Pronounced "O.K. to book" by Dr. All patients and emergency personnel examined for reactions to mace inhalation; see attached. Victims c/o nasal and eye irritation. One patient with asthma admitted to hospital for observation.

This nurse punching out thirty minutes late; requesting overtime. Patient left apparently without aftercare instructions and head injury information. Did not receive needed tetanus immunization.

Suzanne, RN

Note: This nurse received needed tetanus immunization.

MURPHY'S LAW - E.R. NURSING

1. When the patient is ready to go to his room, and the nurse from the floor finally arrives to assist in the transport, the consulting doctor arrives AT THE EXACT MOMENT to do an examination. The nurse leaves, saying, "call when you are ready."

2. When you need a doctor he is:
   a. In the bathroom
   b. On a code
   c. Talking to the tax man, his wife, his ex-wife
   d. Scrubbing for surgery
   e. Flying in a storm over Mexico
   f. The resident was up all night and needs to go back to U.C.L.A. before rounds
   g. In an elevator with the new admissions clerk

3. One hour before change of shift:
   a. The doctor leaves and the county hospital refuses to accept a transfer patient and the NEW doctor refuses to send the patient until he's done a full work-up of his own, add another four hours in the ER
   b. The new doctor is an internist, meticulously and painfully thorough (ie: does not know the secret formula for quick, accurate assessment)
   c. The paramedics bring in a full arrest (CPR IN PROGRESS)
   d. A drunk patient decides to wake up and climb over the side rail and you are responsible for his safety
   e. The police and eight fireman bring in a PCP user - it takes 10 people to hold him down
   f. The new nursing supervisor won't answer her page for more help
   g. A narcotic is found to be missing during the shift-change count
   h. An abnormal lab report is found on a patient who left, and there is no home phone number
   i. You see that the doctor decided to admit someone without telling you. This means at least an hour of work, and the next shift will let you hear about it!

j. Mrs. Jones from the convalescent home needs her bladder tube changed. An emergency?
k. The clerk tells you there is a "nurse call"
l. The Demerol abuser is back at the desk, pounding his fist and yelling loudly
m. The "nurse call" - wants to know what measles looks like and if it resembles Herpes
n. The new doctor yells because his saddle oxfords got dirty
o. A psych patient who has been determined "medically clear" must wait two hours in the emergency room for the ambulance **...**

And the cacophony continues **..........**

MADNESS MADNESS MADNESS

Sometimes you feel as if you are eaten alive by all of the requirements:

Suzanne: Please read this - Jan

CLINICAL NOTEBOOK

A QUICK OVERVIEW OF THE NEW STANDARDS AND GUIDELINES FOR CARDIOPULMONARY RESUSCITATION AND EMERGENCY CARDIAC CARE.

"New standards and guidelines for cardiopulmonary - resuscitation (CPR) and emergency cardiac care (ECC) were recently published in a very complete and lengthy article in the ***Journal of The American Medical Association*** (***JAMA***). The article resulted from the 1985 National Conference on Cardiopulmonary Resuscitation (CPR) and Emergency Cardiac Care (ECC). The following is a review of the highlights of that article, representing changes from the 1980 standards and guidelines. The reader is referred to the original source for more detailed information ... "

Dear Suzanne,

Did you like this article? Important! Remember the required Advanced Cardiac Class next weekend (I know it's your weekend off, I'm sorry - but it is required).

I don't have a current CPR card for you. Also, those classes you requested for continuing education requirements were not approved because they don't relate to your work in the emergency room. When does your license expire?

Jan

The echoes are always with me. Day after day, a drama, a moment of impact **...** The rules and regulations never prepare you.

THE MOVIE

I have been taking my work home with me lately. Too many times. I've awakened in the middle of the night over these faces.

The faces tell me that I'm still alive, still feeling, still vulnerable, and in danger of losing my ability to help. I'm in danger of losing professional distance, armor which keeps me from dissolving into tears, from turning into a casualty rather than a calm and helping presence.

The face I'm remembering is the face of a ten-year-old child. He's been in an auto wreck. One in which his mother dies and he's unscathed. Despite our attempts to save her, she dies. She dies without a mark on her body, but with the word 'no' in her eyes.

I'm seeing the child's face because it is the face of fearful imagining. It is the face surrounded by aunts and uncles and adults who lower their voices and go into the back room. But, they won't let him in, won't let him see, won't let him hear.

A face that asks where is my mother, why is everyone crying, why won't they tell me?

On his face, his ten-year-old face, is a movie, a movie where someone tells him, "You can come in and see you mom, she wants a hug, she's ALRIGHT!" In the movie he kisses her and she wakes up and he's powerful and strong. He's made her smile, he's made her live. But, he is having trouble with the movie because his eyes are seeing the tense and saddened faces of his relatives. His ears are hearing the muffled cries and his forehead is feeling the soft caress of my hand as I look deeply into his eyes now.

I look into his eyes and know that I must speak. I tell them, in the curtained back room:

"The child must know!"

They don't want to hear this. They don't want to tell him.

"Someone must!"

They look at me. The doctor turns his eyes away.

He must be told, otherwise, the movie will continue in his head, and he will make it all his fault. It will become bigger than the car and the ambulance that bore them there. His fantasy will be a giant that has devoured him!

I look into those dark, frightened eyes.

I begin with the truth.

"Your mother loves you very much, can you feel it?"

He nods his head.

The relatives begin to cry.

I feel tears streaming down my face.

I don't know how to continue.

Just then, the priest arrives.

The child says, "My mother is dead."

The priest gathers him in his arms and says, "Yes, Mihijito, your mama has gone to heaven."

And we are crying, we are all crying, and he is the one who is most quiet; we are crying for him.

And now, at four a.m., I hope that this movie which awakens me will end soon. Soon.

These frames of life and death spark remembrances of all of us who give care. We had a parent, sibling, spouse, child ... they call us to reach within ourselves and find our greatest tool: compassion.

In the dark hour of this child, I can say, with pride, I was there, and it mattered.

BATTLES

One of the best doctors I ever worked with saw how much I took it all to heart. He said, "Suzanne, you must learn to relax, and it will all get done if you first stop and take a deep breath. I see you wearing your body like a brace, holding yourself together like someone in a vise. Soon your muscles will give in, your gut will bleed. Put yourself in a mental bubble as you carry out your actions. Do what is needed, but allow yourself to breathe."

That same doctor held me tight as I cried over the death of a child. He held me until my breaths were even, calm.

In times of severe stress, I remember him, remember to breathe. A dead nurse is no help at all.

Another doctor gave me good advice. "Choose your battles." he said. So I learned to know what I could live with, in this room of rooms.

On one occasion I said to him, "I want you to explain to that patient what you are doing. He deserves to know."

"I just told him."

"He's not satisfied and it will save problems later."

His expression changed from annoyance to humor; "You've chosen!" he said, going to the patient's room.

We will have to laugh or we will cry.

THE DOCTOR

The doctor, a resident at the university who is moonlighting here tonight, (he could be kicked out of the resident program if he's caught) lies asleep in the doctor's room.

He's been with patients at the clinic all day; this night, he's trying to catch a couple of hours of sleep before grand rounds at 8 a.m.

He's been mean, cranky, demanding. STAT this, STAT that.

"You're going to STAT yourself right out of a nurse!" my co-worker tells him.

He growls. "I'm the doctor and you'll do what I say!"

She smiles sweetly without comment.

The pace slows. He goes to his room to sleep.

Now he snores, unshaven, exhausted.

The nurse puts a wet, warm cloth in his outstretched hand. A dark stain forms on his crotch.

FROM MY JOURNAL

There once was a nurse named Sue
Who always knew what to do.
She took out a dipstick
(She thought it was lipstick)
And painted her lips ketone blue.

WHERE DO I STAND

Some call taking a stand insubordination. Others call it a nurse's duty, in line with the Nurse Practice Act. I ask myself where I stand on the issues: abortion, surrogate motherhood, gene engineering, euthanasia? There are so many sides to consider - our technology is running ahead of us, we are not ready for the leap. We are often caught off guard ... for example, terminal illness. Who defines quality of life? Is an E.E. G. (brain wave test) a true indicator of that quality? It is a true sign of the meaning of that life? Do we judge those lives in dollars and cents? And WHEN are the decisions made?

Euthanasia, active: take a life. Euthanasia, passive: Refrain from prolonging life. No heroics.

I took care of a baby.
I took care of a baby.
The baby gasped for breath.
The baby was blue
he was thin and his eyes were blue.
He struggled with his every breath;
Terminal, he won't last a year.
He struggled for his every breath, his whole body clenching,
giving a cry, as if his whole being were a heart itself.
Knowing what it wanted.

"The baby should die. He has no chance." said the doctor, knowing of the infant's terminal illness.

(The baby still struggled, clenching, eyes wide. He'd made his choice).

"He should be allowed to die in peace." said the hesitant doctor.

One hour, two hours went by; the baby fought; his eyes met mine. He didn't cry, he only lived, in the way that we all must live. The spark proceeding, continuing, choosing. Against all odds. Fighting. There was a determination in his fight. Heroic.

The heart began to tire. The gasps grew fainter, a whisper of his message.

"Why do we have to prolong the agony of his life?" moaned the doctor, as the IV dripped, the heart rate began to slow.

"Doctor, he's tiring. I'm afraid he'll code any minute."

"I don't want to tube him."

"Doctor, are you going to tube him or not?"

The small spark continued.

"So we can run up a huge bill, and the parents have to pay, and the baby will die anyway?"

The babe was no longer crying, but still he fought, clenched his little fists, as if it were his only fight. There was no fear in his eyes, only determination. He had no fear; that was OUR domain. The baby spoke in grunts. If ever a heart wanted beating ...

"Doctor, listen. You have to do something ... Doctor, what are you going to do?????"

The doctor pulled at his hair, groaned, "Oh, God, I'm not GOD!"

"The paramedics brought him in. They couldn't stand to watch him struggle. Look, he's fighting so hard. He's not ready to _____."

"Damn, damn the law suits, the blame, the high costs of malpractice insurance ... where is the dignity, where is the peace?"

"Doctor, what are you going to do? He wants to stay."

Doctor, where do you stand? Nurse, where do you stand? Patient, where do you stand?

Right now, this moment, we are suffering, we are all suffering. (We used to know. Once, we all knew, and lived what we knew, when to begin, when to end, when to keep, when to release ...).

I thought I saw thanks in those eyes;
if ever there was a soul, I was meeting it,
if ever there was a purpose, I was attending it,
and with the softer rhythm of his tubed breaths,
his blue eyes finally closed in rest.

Until the next time.
Until it WAS time.

MORE JOURNAL

4 a.m. again. A day off. I have worked five twelve-hour shifts in a row. Rest. Laundry. Time with my kids. The youngest is "acting out," he has bitten another child and the parents are threatening to sue. When did lawsuits begin to seep into our everyday lives as solutions? I now carry malpractice insurance (and car insurance, rent insurance, etc.) as if it were a guarantee against the pain and suffering of life.

No groceries. Get up and go. I'll tell them a bedtime story tonight; probably go to bed at 8:30. I'm so tired!

Now that S. is moving out and I am no longer seeing the 'doctor' who helped me make the transition ... I feel so empty. Where is the partner who can love me AND my children, who can understand me? I feel as if I am always helping others - who will nurture me, the strong one, the one who does it all? Am I asking too much? Don't know what I do wrong; can't seem to get them to appreciate me. Do I give too much? Do I smother them? Or, I'm so tired that I can't even cook a meal ...

5:30 a.m. I can't believe I just agreed to work today. J. called in sick again. Don't know how he functions, so much booze. Day care closed today, get a sitter. There goes movie money. I'll tell them a story tonight ...

7:30 p.m. When will I learn to say no ...!

DISCIPLINE OR OPPRESSION?

SUBJECT: Dress Code

Recently, it has become necessary to remind employees of this hospital policy of professional dress.

NURSES:

White uniforms must be worn. Pants allowed, if tailored and loose-fitting. No T-type shirts or ruffles may be worn. Earrings may be simple and close to the ears; no dangling or HAZARDOUS styles. Nail polish clear or light pink. Hair short or off the collar. Scrub suits in areas allowed, emergency, surgery, and OB only. Navy blue or white sweaters or white lab jackets only, no print or stripe coverings.

Shoes must be comfortable with rubber soles; no open toes or clog-type styles.

Men may wear mustaches trimmed and neat; no long hair.

Nylons may be tan or white only; stockings must be worn.

Thank you for your cooperation.

Dear Suzanne,

I must remind you to clock in and out at the appropriate times. I'll have to dock your pay if you're seven minutes late. Also, you can't punch in late and work later to make up the difference. Remember that the schedule is made out a month ahead of time. Please put schedule requests in writing and make a copy for the nursing office. Also, my records show that you need to come to the fire class. How about next Monday? I know it's your day off, but it's required.

Thanks,

Jan

P.S. We're having a disaster drill next week and you are scheduled. Look at the manual.

WE HAVE NO EMPATHY FOR EACH OTHER ...

SISTERS

We have been mandated by the Nursing Practice Act to be accountable for our choices. We are told by physicians that we are not educated enough to make decisions. Administrators require us to follow rules and regulations but abandon us when we need support. The media ignores us except to make judgments about our sexual practices.

The public does not see us unless we make a mistake, or do not do what "should" have been done despite medical hierarchy and hospital policy. We are required to take continuing education classes at considerable expense, often the same classes which physicians take. We make 1/4 of what physicians make - yet we fill in the gaps which doctors have left by going into specialties and leaving families without "family doctors." We are a separate but equally important discipline. Here, in the tiny nurse's lounge, (which is really an alcove between the utility room and the medicine room), we VENTILATE:

NURSE A: "My feet are killing me! I've just spent $50.00 on a pair of uniform shoes and my feet feel like they have been encased in cement!"

NURSE B: "I just bought two uniforms and it cost me $64.00. A patient puled on me the first day I wore one."

NURSE A: "Did you get your raise?"

NURSE B: "You mean my dollar an hour a year?"

NURSE A: "What happened to your decision to take more classes? Are you still going for your degree?"

NURSE B: "They told me I'd make a hundred dollars more a year ... New grads make only slightly less than I make after ten years ..."

NURSE A: "I just got malpractice insurance. Ever since Joanie was sued - the doctor refused to see a patient and she let the patient go. He needed a CT scan. The doctor said it wasn't necessary. The patient had a seizure and a respiratory arrest. They claimed SHE was responsible for the patient getting proper care ...

PATIENTS LIE

The following story indicates a pattern which began for me and which again signaled burnout. It describes the kind of situation which can happen despite the best intentions of many who provide care ... yet I took it personally, as if I were at fault, somehow defective ...

He SAID: "My girlfriend bit my tongue."

True enough, the tongue was swollen in the wide, blank face. Something in me should have warned: in retrospect, there was a glassiness to his eyes, and didn't he smell of urine? But he was walking steadily, if not lumbering - a big man - to the stretcher. Couldn't fit altogether on the narrow gurney. The side rails had to remain down. I didn't heed my inner warning. He didn't fit ... he looked O.K., we were busy ...

The doctor said, "I'll stitch that tongue, get me the cocaine" (to stop the bleeding).

Routine: inject the wound, let it numb, suture.

Meanwhile: room two - chest pain, hook him up to the monitor, get an EKG; room two-B, vomiting, grab a towel ...

CRASH BANG!

The big man, flopping in the middle of the floor, arm flailing against the metal tray (suture material everywhere) his head hitting the floor.

My inner voice said: "I SHOULD HAVE THOUGHT SEIZURE! WHY DIDN'T I THINK SEIZURE?"

The doctor slides beneath him, cradling his head (he's too heavy to lift), two nurses bend over his flailing arms, trying to start an IV to give him needed anti-seizure medicine ... a woman respiratory therapist, tries to

(WHY DIDN'T I THINK SEIZURE?)

give him an oxygen mask, her great breasts leaning over his face as she offers. (HE SAID HIS GIRLFRIEND BIT HIS TONGUE ...)

Two passing policemen with a pre-book patient.

The man begins to awaken in confused agitation.

NOW he is punching with fists, trying to shake loose of the doctor's safety headlock. The nurses are riding his thighs to keep him form yanking his newly placed "lines," tubes with life-giving, presence-gaining medicine. His broken tongue spits blood and spatters everyone. The police men come to firmly "engage" him, and as the anticonvulsant is now being given, the hospital administrator strolls into the bloody, insane mess and registers, like a cartoon imbecile, to the jerking humping, flailing,

"What the ... "

(I SHOULD HAVE THOUGHT SEIZURE ...)

The medicine takes effect. One by one, we all recoil, wrinkled, blood-spattered, immodest (uniforms hunched above buttocks, below brassieres) - from the lunatic scene. There are more patients, still they arrive, get a gown, get a scrub suit, admit the poor man to the hospital, fill out an incident report (EXACT LOCATION ...)

I'm sorry, we must laugh. Patients lie, and WE are caught out. Yes, I'll fill out an incident report.

(I CAN'T BELIEVE I DIDN'T THINK SEIZURE ...)

(This happened before we knew much about AIDS)

JOURNAL 4 a.m. ANOTHER PANIC ATTACK

Such a stupid mistake, not even thinking of seizure. It's as though something in me short-circuited. We were busy, but I should have thought ...

And my son, still acting out. I'm a failure as a mother. Never mind as a lover. I give and give, and all of it ends this way, always. No time to see my friends, no time to take a class (except nursing, mandatory), God, I'm trapped!

I used to draw, paint. One of my teachers wanted my painting, said I'd be known one day. Then marriage, moving, no more art. Exceptional an occasional sketch, between meals.

I wrote. My poem won a prize, was read by the girl with the long blond braid. I heard people sighing as she spoke.

I read. Discussions on world affairs keep me interested; another nurse at work calls me Nurse Deep. God, I'm so damned serious. Why can't I laugh ... Still not sleepy. Five a.m. comes too soon ...

ABUSE HAS MANY FACES

"You bitch! I want pain medicine now!"

"Sir, I know you are in pain, but the doctor must see you first. And, swearing at ME is not necessary."

"I'm sorry, this fucking headache is killing me!" (Tears. Arms over eyes. Moans. Darken room. Cool cloth to head).

"You're such a nice nurse."

"This will sting a bit."

"What is it?" The needle darts its way through thick, scarred, pale flesh. The scars of numerous injections.

"Demerol."

"How much?"

"Fifty milligrams."

"I need seventy-five milligrams."

"The doctor ordered fifty."

"Tell him I need more."

"I'll ask him."

(Clenched fists, sullen face).

"I'm sorry, that's all he will order.

(Up in a flash, over the railing).

"You fucking bitch!" he said running out the door.

The doctor looks at recent charts which show that the patient has been here twice in the last week. He writes "drug-seeking behavior" on the chart. We can't confront the patient about this, lest we are charged with "slander."

Bitch. Truth or slander?

Dear Clara Barton, of the dark cape, noble brow, of the calm dignity, I need you. Rescue me, come to my aid, I am in distress.

I hold the dark bird.

FIVE

MALAISE

Long, arduous hours. Little acknowledgment. Militaristic or arbitrary rules and regulations. High drama, with extreme highs and lows, the feeling of never being enough. Growing up with alcoholism allows one to accept, even crave, this way of life. Being on the edge which is certainly part of being in the Emergency Room, keeps the adrenaline flowing, keeps one feeling "alive."

At home, a love-hate relationship kept me up, often into early morning hours, in a pattern not unlike that which my parents shared for 17 years. My partner often found fault with the relationship, usually late at night, and "discussions" would ensue. Yet, when I tired of this pattern, and agreed with him, that maybe we should separate, he would say "don't leave me."

Something had to give.

The Center for Disease Control now calls it CFS, or, Chronic Fatigue Syndrome. It started with a flu which wouldn't get better. It left me ill with swollen glands, low-grade fever, pharyngitis, irritable bowel, sudden weight gain, and difficulty concentrating. And the worst symptom: debilitating fatigue.

In 1986, it was a new disease. Today we are no closer to understanding its cause. For two years, attempting to live with it, live with the stigma around it, live with decreased abilities, and still deal with the Emergency Room, my relationship, my children - left little room for pondering. I was hanging on by my fingernails. It was a disaster. It was also the beginning of a message which, like the echoes in the abandoned hallways on my first assignment as a nurse frightened and stilled me. Life is more than this. Life is more than mere survival. Life is more than suffering, surviving, getting through the shift. The illness was my body telling me to pay attention.

I went to per-diem work, still attempting to do it all, and still dealing with the issues.

PATIENT ADVOCATE

The doctor, who is new, tells her, "It's just the flu, go home and rest." He's with one of these new H.M.O.'s, a board member. I have seen the lab report: the white count is elevated, and the amylase is too. Very elevated. Dangerously so.

"What about these lab results?" I ask him, privately.

"Nothing to worry about." he says.

A patient with another insurance plan would most definitely be admitted, I know. I also know that with pancreatitis, the patient should not eat. Doing so would put the pancreas under stress. Intravenous fluids are important. The doctor tells her none of this.

I pull him aside and ask him about the high amylase. "Nothing we can't handle at home, doctors tend to admit patients too readily." he says, walking away.

It's true, many hospital admissions occur out of fear of lawsuit. And, home health care is becoming an effective, safe way to render care. But, this isn't one of those situations. This patient needs close observation by trained people. I am sure that she will have to pull teeth with THIS doctor and THIS plan to get a nurse to see her at home.

I take a deep breath and tell her, out of his hearing range. "You did not hear this from me. You have the right to ask questions until you are satisfied. You have the right to a second opinion. I can give you the referral of someone I trust, if you would like. Write it down yourself, because I will deny it if I am asked."

Many of the patients who have signed up for this particular HMO are Medicare patients who have signed over their Medicare benefits to the company. Many do not know that they can DIS-enroll - and - think they have to put up with such poor care. Like this little old lady:

She was brought to the emergency room with an obviously broken humerus. The right upper arm bent outward a good two inches above the elbow. She had sustained a fall, and the paramedics brought her to us, the nearest facility, which they are required by LAW to do. While keeping her arm in a sling, assessing vital signs and circulation distal to the break (below it), to make sure that the pulse was unimpaired (broken bones can interfere with the free flow of blood to the tissues, causing necrosis and compromising the appendage), and checking the feel of the skin (coolness indicates such a compromise), the clerk did what she must do; she called the physician advisor of the HMO. The poor old lady was in obvious pain, but we could not give her anything until X-rays were done to confirm the break, and to determine if it needed to be surgically corrected.

We were inhibited from doing ANYTHING to make this lady comfortable, when, over the phone, the doctor refused authorization for us to treat the lady. He admonished us to tell her to go the THEIR facility, several miles away.

The poor lady had no transportation, lived alone.

The ER doctor looked at it briefly and ascertained that she was not at risk to travel, and, at our hospital expense, and to her great discomfort, the lady was given a cab voucher. She was forced to travel in a cab - still in pain, and at considerable risk of movement of the arm, despite the sling. (Pain medications which can alter consciousness cannot be given unless supervision will follow).

In another instance, a patient is told to see her private doctor the next day. The HMO doctor has refused further tests. In effect, tying the ER doctor's hands. She is old, she has no relatives to help her. Her condition is such that she might need to be admitted, (a borderline condition) if she had another plan. She does not. The social worker is off duty. I go to the doctor and tell her the situation.

"I'm not a social worker," says the doctor.

I escort the patient to her care, admonishing her to return if needed. There has been nothing any of us can do.

While I am an advocate of *care* which is effectively managed, most insurance plans allow for emergency treatment and leave the admission to the physician in that instance. This doctor would have admitted this patient if the HMO doctor had not refused.

These people are "falling through the cracks." "Universal" coverage must be made available, as an adjunct to employment-based plans, to include persons who have fallen out of the system, or who have no access (illegal, unemployed).

WRITTEN ON A SCRAP OF PAPER (Again, at 4 a.m.):

SOLUTIONS: (radical) Start at source. Physicians should be required to take courses which deal with patient needs IN TOTAL, not just the body. Be REQUIRED to intern as nurses. Same duties. Same considerations. Should have to stay at the bedside, perform baths, do continuing head to toe assessments. LEARN ABOUT RESOURCES AVAILABLE to help the total patient.

Nurses should have free medical care!

Insurance Companies: Promote health rather than illness. Reimburse prevention as being cost-effective, provided the "prevention" is based on sound premises. Acknowledge and give recompense for Nursing Services. In the hospital, instead of penalizing patients for a poor hospital management, insurance companies should communicate with physicians in a way that they will understand effective management, rather than doing what's "always been done" as treatment.

Since most hospitalization are driven by physician order, it should be physicians who are penalized if they are not willing to learn about patient care management. They need to learn to consider the questions:

* *ARE THERE REASONS WHY THE CARE BEING GIVEN CANNOT BE DONE IN AN OUTPATIENT SETTING?*

* *HOW CAN WE BEST RETURN THE PATIENT TO OPTIMUM HEALTH?*

Too many physicians are concerned only with what's in front of them, and have no concept of, or desire to understand, discharge planning, let alone the psychological and spiritual aspects of care. A multi-discipline effort must be rewarded by insurance companies.

H.M.O.'s: Could be managed by nurse practitioners with physicians handling complex cases and writing prescriptions. Prescription writing by nurses is being studied now. Nurses have a broad breadth and scope of knowledge and if Physician Assistants, whose training is shorter and more technician-focused, can write prescriptions, nurses are certainly capable of doing so under specific circumstances.

HMO physicians should give full credit to physicians who are with patients in the emergency rooms, or else should come and see the patient. Telephone assessment AT THIS STAGE is a blatant breech of medical ethics. The doctor with the patient in the emergency room should make the decisions for initial, pre-admission care.

Patients/Clients: TAKE RESPONSIBILITY FOR YOUR BODIES!! STOP BEING LAZY! Learn the medicines you take. Ask questions. Learn to take temperatures. Take antibiotics until they are FINISHED, unless you have a bad reaction to them. Then, let your doctor know! And, know your allergies. If you can't remember them, make a list. Think of the health worker as your PARTNER IN HEALTH, not a God. Remember, you have the right to ask, a right to know. A right to say no, to ask why.

Oh, God, I can hear the uproar. I feel naughty, guilty. I feel alone. Why? BECAUSE I AM.

Instead of protesting, one loud voice, nurses give in. To safety violations, to ethical violations (don't speak of it, let the administrators decide), to our own perfectionism, and the inability to say no. To taking the blame - to intimidation:

"Due to the number of patient complaints, you might not get your bonus this quarter."

No one asked about the complaints, or followed them up. Or, asked OUR side. For example:

A man who is capable of doing so says, "wipe me." I tell him, "do it yourself."

A woman who is uncomfortable, (and about whom I have been PLEADING with technicians and doctor to get things in motion), wants to be taken off an uncomfortable back board. But she has been in a traffic accident, and we must consider a possible spinal injury, until it is cleared.

I've been burned. I once took a patient off a board when a physician decided not to order an X-ray assessment. He hadn't "cleared the cervical spine but said, in a cavalier way, that it was "alright." The patient complained of numbness in the hand. When I told the doctor and he THEN ordered an X-ray, the first thing he said, when he found out there was a fracture, "the nurse took him off the board."

But this old lady is miserable. She yells at me: "Do IT NOW!"

My breath catches. This isn't fair. She doesn't know the fight I have been conducting on her behalf, that there is only one overworked X-ray technician.

"I am doing the best I can and I am here to help you but I am not here to have you yell at me. I say. She says I am rude.

I wonder if it is rude to stand up for yourself once in a while? But, I feel guilty because she is old and uncomfortable. I leave the room in silence. When I return, when the test is done and the X-ray cleared, she says, "I am sorry, nurse."

I kiss her cheek and hold her hand. "Let's get you off that hard ol' board," I tell her.

The nurse cannot win in these circumstances. If the doctor doesn't do what is needed, or doesn't know, we are at risk of lawsuit if that choice results in patient harm. Nurses have been found responsible, in legal determinations, for not obtaining the proper care for the patient. Many physicians do not understand this concept.

Once (later), when working at a prominent cosmetic surgeon's office, I was severely reprimanded and labeled "recalcitrant" (in writing) when I informed a physician that I was uncomfortable administering a strong sedative/analgesic to a patient who was going to drive after the two-hour procedure. The office had had a former patient who had driven himself to the airport and "woke-up" on the plane, not knowing how he got there. Still, this physician insisted that I "follow orders," had a tantrum, yelled and hit walls, and acted generally crazy. His shaking hands and emotional lability made me fear for his patients. The head physician backed <u>him</u>, not me, despite legal advisement which had been issued and stated that certain procedures were not to be done unless the patient had a ride home. Another example of nurse-in-the-middle between the "pecking" order, patient rights, and licensure considerations.

It gives me physical pain to have to fight to get things done. I hate confrontations. But I have been burned. Once, a doctor ordered Demerol for a woman who had been in an accident. I said that her pressure was too low and that she might need surgery. The doctor insisted, "Don't worry, she's in pain, go ahead and give it."

I gave it, against my better judgment - and was proven uncomfortably right: her pressure bottomed, she "passed out," and we had to work feverishly with fluids and oxygen to bring her pressure back to a normal status. During this time the doctor said, (like being cut out of a cookie cutter) "the nurse gave her some Demorol and she went out."

I resolved never again to go against this voice inside. It is BETRAYAL, nothing less, for a physician to do this. It is a toxic power game which is meant to keep nurses off balance, squashed. *Nurses, if your learn nothing else, learn to trust your gut!*

When a decision is made to change something, it is as if the forces that be want to test one's determination. When a people who have been invisible take steps to be heard, they are put down shot-down, even, or especially, by those whose own ranks have gone along with the status quo. But as we have seen, the system is rupturing, the stresses have become too many, and the truth is leaking out all over: THE SYSTEM NEEDS HELP!

It is hard for me to speak up. Those words are on the page and they have, for the most part, until now, been private words. Like many nurses, I have my own inner "Wicked Witch" who says, who do you think you are, to say such things?" and "everyone will hate you for saying this," and "watch out, you're going to offend someone." And so I stew and fret some more. I am stuck. I am still propelled by the needs of the patients, but hate the conundrum.

I want to stop: where is the grace. Grant me a healing attitude, God ... I must go on, I can't quit now ...

THE EYE

blink
eye
blink
eye
southward northward
dart sleep eye sleep
the
eye of the soul still
moves me
I wake in
dread I want morning
the shadows, gut rumbles want morning ...

in the wedge of sky
between buildings
the blue
between
the roofs and windows
it searches for
the yellow-over-blue
wants
the hours
sofa chair cat jumbled
books, pink brocade over
closed
eyelids in the sun
sweet veined grace

I HOLD THE DARK BIRD

Junkie, they bring you. Dark to your surroundings, to the year, to your name. To your breath reeking of stale alcohol and kisses gone dry. To your hair matted with street grit, to your cheeks bearing traces - capillary maps - of daily binges, to your nose, a resort for street "snow."

John Doe.

You've done it all, you bear the marks. Here, tattooed, the tail of a peacock, once proud, dragging on your wasted forearm. There, a mermaid's sagging breasts, her tail full of many-eyed scales, needle marks in each.

Unseeing eyes, seeking heaven.

We wear gloves because you are so dirty. We make faces because you smell. Though you are young, you wear an old man's clothes: brown stained pants, thrift-store shirt, oversized shoes. You carry a lighter with a "playboy" insignia, mockery of the man you once were or could never be. The other nurses call you Scumbag. Dirtball.

I wonder about you. I wonder what belly-laughs you gave as a child, only to receive scowls, lashings of an impoverished hand. Or maybe you had everything, excess, made too many excuses, got away with too much. Or maybe it was destiny, or maybe you just took wrong turns until, suddenly, you are here.

You are freeze-dried potential. And I, with my white clad legs, with my junk in my pocket (nurse packet, scissors, pen, watch, tape, armmonia spirits) - I have it together. I am equipped to soothe you, FIX you, release you.

But I am soothing now more by rote than by feel. I, who was taught to be a nice person, to be "good," to give, to be polite, polite at all costs, am confronted with you.

You make me angry, with your potential. I think, but for the grace of God, I might be on that stretcher. But, for some spark, (or for that polite socialization), I too, might have huddled in dark corners. I, too, have felt lonely, bereft, helpless. Still, I want to condemn you, ridicule you, get you out of my emergency room as soon as possible, for your weakness is NEED, and mine, I am learning, is Being Needed. And I can't help you.

We give you a drug to counteract the narcotic, a drug which closes heaven's gateway, the dope-bound endorphin receptor, so that you awaken with a start, and shiver, and sweat, and shiver some more. Lucky.

I make notations on the chart, avoid you with clenched jaw and braced shoulders (together, together), my nurturing will be in vain. I am right; once better, you growl and sign out against medical advice (the drug we gave could wear off, the next 'hit' could be your last), afraid to stay for fear of arrest, denying, even as the last molecule of medicine reaches your pleasure center, that it was anything but beer. NO HERO IN HEROIN.

You mumble and avert your eyes and dart off into the street to find the 'friends' who abandoned you at the doorstep.

I know that one day you will probably return, possible blue and damp and cold and limp and breathless. And, God help me, I'll probably be waiting. Keeping it together, Trying to help.

* * * * * * * * *

Dear Suzanne,

"Such a pleasure to hear from you. It sounds as though you've been very busy and successful. I am saddened to hear of your discouragement. We need good nurses so badly. It is a shame when the system becomes so overwhelming. Ultimately, it is the patient who suffers."

I have written to one of my nursing instructors. I keep at it. I am still touched by the patients, as they come in, with their pain, with their statements about existence. I am deeply moved by their realization that what I see and participate in is indeed, a privilege. The brief moments of transcendence are fewer and fewer, compared to the frustration of - no, the TOXICITY of "the system." Is there, as Sartre said, "No exit?" What are we doing?

SOMETHING OFF THE WALL

Been thinking about you, old man. Attempted suicide. Living in an old folk's home, but sound of mind. Only, God's wrath, old.

"They lied to me. They said if I took it, I'd die and I didn't die, and they lied. What do you want to go and save me for? I'm old, no one wants me. My children are too busy, haven't got time for me. I had a friend, a lady friend, only last week she died, and now I got nobody. I want to die!"

Oh, what do I say to you, old man, what do I say? I can't tell you it will get better. I can't tell you that your family wants you. I can't tell you that it doesn't hurt. I can't tell you that I have felt the same way.

All I can think to say is something off the wall. "I think you are probably a very wonderful person."

You are quiet, and I don't know if I, who usually say the right thing (I've always been told I'm a good listener) or the therapeutic thing (from my brief trial as a psychiatric nurse last spring) have indeed said what I needed. Or, should I have spoken at all? MY INTUITION SEEMS TO BE FAILING.

I look for the expression on your face which says I have eased the pain ... and suddenly realize that this is how I felt when Daddy didn't come home, and Mommy was worrying, and I was a failure at being a daughter, otherwise I could have cheered her up.

GET A GRIP SUZANNE! I tell myself. But the messenger doesn't stop until the message is delivered.

I am a wounded healer, working in a wounded system. It will take me more time to understand what that means to me as a nurse, as part of the whole. The echo grows deeper: it is a harrowing call.

BLACK GLOVE

"Where d'ya want this one?"

The small dark-haired cop drags one in. Black. Hog-tied. I notice a few abrasions on his face. The left cheek looks swollen.

I wonder what the man did and why he's hog-tied. Probably PCP. But he doesn't have that bulging look, the look and strength which accompanies the effects of the tranquilizer. He's too placid. And there are only two cops with him; usually it takes eight or so. And he's pale; PCP-ers usually have that about-to-stroke redness to the face. No, not PCP.

I point to the "holding room," where we put psych patients, pre-books, and maternity patients, (hopefully not all at once!).

"Be there in a moment," I tell the cop. He's slight, slim, and, I notice wearing one black glove.

"What's that for?" I ask another nurse.

"Oh, they say he gets tough out in the field, anybody gives him lip."

When I get to the room, the patient is still hog-tied, stomach down on the gurney. He's sullen. The cop shoves him, whacks him in the head.

"Hello, sir," I say, "what's wrong today?"

The man blinks, lowers his head.

The little cop shoves him, grabs him by the shirt. "Answer the nurse, man." the cop's lip is drawn down, his teeth are clenched. He shoves again, causing the man to wince.

The man mumbles.

"Speak up, man!" says the cop shoving him again.

"I'm going to take your blood pressure and give you a shot for the cut, then the doctor will stitch it." I turn to the cop and tell him that he doesn't need to keep up the rough stuff, since the man is hog-tied. I leave, but when I come back with the bowl of betadine and the sponge, the cop is shoving him again.

I decide to call the watch commander, telling him about the one black glove, and what I have been told. The watch commander responds, "He's been told about that."

Later, I hear that the cop has been suspended. I don't know if it is because of my call, or if it is because the one black glove has, like the willful alter-self in *Dr. Strangelove*, betrayed him.

Many years later - about ten - this same policeman is on national television defending his deeds, captured on video film, as he joins three other policeman in the beating of a down and "tazered" suspect. He asserts that he was the odd one out, trying to keep them form beating the suspect further. Methinks the man doth protest too much.

DO THE RIGHT THING

A Pediatrician who is on duty in the emergency room is about to send a "cash" patient to another facility. The child is feverish, has belly pain, has been vomiting. He has been sick most of the day, and he is dehydrated, which shows in his lab work. Further, he has a shift in his white cells which is a classic sign of appendicitis.

But, he is a cash patient, and the doctor (who has "stock" in this hospital) does not want to incur costs, knowing that the dollars will never be seen. This is a scenario which repeats itself hundreds of times in hospitals all over Southern California and other areas which have a large illegal immigrant population. It hasn't been resolved, and needs to be considered, now, some ten years later.

Still, I know that the risk for lawsuit is great, that if the boy goes out in a care, without medical aid, the appendix could rupture. Further, I would not want my son to be treated in this way. The doctor is preparing to send him out and I can't stand it. I tell him that we are taking a big risk, what if something happens?

The doctor fumes and fusses, but admits the child who later goes to surgery when the appendix does rupture. The doctor says to me, "Are you happy now?" - but doesn't acknowledge that we in all probability saved ourselves from a gigantic lawsuit, not to mention that we did the right thing.

"If you must err," said my teacher, "do it on the side of the patient, and you won't go wrong."

Our poor, sick, complicated system is cracking up over scenes such as these, and it's getting worse.

We must give good care, we can be sued for not doing so; we are confronted with patients in this community who cannot pay for it, or for insurance.

One physician I worked with had the habit of telling poor patients to sign out "against medical advice," so that if anything happened, the "legal" document would take him off the hook. When I questioned this practice, he said "Suzanne, don't make my life miserable."

These doctors are not bad people. In fact, most are good physicians who have allowed themselves to get stuck in the dollars-and-cents dilemma of health care. This is not without good reason. More and more patients use emergency rooms as clinics, because they do not have, or do not qualify for, medical insurance. The public facilities are full to the brim. Local hospitals must take their turn in accepting indigent patients. But, some physicians who are on staff for hospitals simply do not take call, or become difficult to find when it is their turn to take call. They don't want to get "stuck" with a non-paying patient.

Many patients take advantage of this, reneging on their responsibilities. The answer will come from all sectors INCLUDING NURSES, when they put their heads together to solve this. People need good care, but people also need to take more responsibility. Still, the situations sometimes get out of hand. Regardless of the outcome of these questions, we must put the patients first.

Another physician with whom I worked was severely burned out, as I was becoming, and had developed a hatred for the "dregs" of society. He especially did not like alcoholics. When one came in one day, he took it upon himself to shove an Ewald tube down the man's nostril. This is a fat red tube used when pumping the stomach of toxic contents. His argument for doing so was that alcohol was a toxin and he did not want to be sued if the patient had taken an overdose.

The angry force with which he actually shoved the tube down the patients nose caused immediate bleeding and the patient, after suction, intravenous lines, monitoring and restraints, as he was now wide awake, needed to be admitted to ICU. When I told the physician that I was fed-up with him taking his hostility out on the patients and to change his attitude, he GRABBED MY ARM and said, "You had better change yours."

When I reported this to the head nurse, who was MALE, I was told, "Boy you're being bitchy today."

In a dysfunctional environment, we are expected to keep our mouths shut, our perceptions are rendered invalid (you're being bitchy, or too sensitive or recalcitrant), and we are either patronized, or reprimanded for our "rebelliousness." The irony for me personally is that I have always (and to my detriment) been a "good girl." A polite person, one who obeys. Given these kinds of "rules" - whether in a household or in a hospital - it is not difficult to see why one is at risk for "burnout."

Earlier I described how some women physicians act as if nurses are peons, not partners in care. One WOMAN doctor I worked with had a habit of throwing orders at us (if we were female; she flirted with the male nurses), and having temper tantrums if we didn't move fast enough for her. She came into the unit searching for something to be wrong - and usually found it. My co-workers and I handled this woman one of two ways - either we avoided her or sucked up and giggled and played the favorites game. In two years of association with this specialist, never once did she call me, or any other nurse by name, first or last. She simply came in, wrote or barked her orders, smooched with the patients, and left.

On one occasion, her child was injured. I cared for the child through X-rays, blood pressure checks, gave needed pain medication, applied ice. Never once did this doctor thank me, or even acknowledge me.

She had a habit, when really angry, of unwrapping her long hair, which she kept in a bun. She would twist it during her tirade, then, when coming to the end of her tantrum, fling the hair in the opposite direction, and re-wrap it, all in the course of about two minutes. Women against each other, power games, erosion of empathy ... hospitals still allow it, and we can no longer afford it.

The majority of health care workers in this country are women. The majority are nurses. We care about the patients, we fight for them. We work overtime for them, and question orders which might harm them. Yet, as a collective group, we are notorious for having no backbone. Some of us prefer to "look out for the patients." But, allowing poor practices to continue does not help patients. It enables a sick system to continue.

Nurses who are self-supporting are at odds with those who have a partner. Issues which the business world has long since dealt with - problems such as child care and pay imbalances (veteran nurses only make a small amount more than new grads) - continue unresolved.

Nurses are still working without lunch breaks, working overtime, and being threatened with charges of patient abandonment if they don't. Problems such as short-staffing and forcing nurses to take dangerously heavy patient loads, again, with the threat of charges of patient abandonment, continue.

What ensues is an "us against them" approach. This leaves nurses to fight each other by gossiping, fighting, triangling against each other. This leaves us powerless and ineffective to make changes.

The media has been no help. Due to the hostility of the women's movement for "traditional" women's roles, nursing has been scorned by some women in a position to help. In discussions of important issues, the medical world is seen as being inhabited by physicians only. Tune in to any program about the state of health care today, and see if any nurses are consulted.

This was illustrated in a way which was right there, for all the nation to see, in brilliant color. None other than Ted Koppel, the celebrated commentator of "Night Line," had a panel of experts on his program to discuss the medical woes which plague us today. On that panel was Lucille Joel, a distinguished nurse and national nursing spokesperson. Ms. Joel was asked not one question, and did not have one opportunity to make any statements whatsoever!

Nurses are solution-seekers. Nurses are an untapped resource for positive change. Hospitals would benefit in abandoning the authoritarian approach for one of "empowerment." Let nurses administer, form ethics committees, develop ways to honor those who are the primary source of help, and then watch that facility turn into a source of inspiration. In so doing, other personnel, so vital to the functioning of a hospital would also be inspired. Let those who would excel do so. Invite the feedback of everyone, including housekeeping services. The wastefulness of our system does not begin and end with dollars and cents! The revitalization of our facilities could happen with a small shift in outlook, with a commitment to respectfulness.

In my dreams?

SIX

RECOVERY

Like my own mother, who was raised by an alcoholic grandmother, I learned behaviors which allowed me to survive, but, which contributed to emotional pain in adult life. Had my mother known about Alanon, we might have begun recovery earlier. She did choose therapy, to deal both with the "wreckage of her past," and the chaotic life of living with an alcoholic. My father was not to blame for his disease, but he was responsible for being in denial. An alcoholic is not a down-in-the gutter drunk, but rather, one whose intake of the chemical leaves others around him (or her) in misery. As the sole breadwinner for many years, he lost jobs because of his drinking. He would disappear , often on a weekend, usually after a martini lunch, only to call at 3 a.m. from a bar in the city, wanting to find his way home.

The rent and bills didn't get paid. My mother, whose tools for detachment were lacking, would obsess, become hysterical, and when he did return, be both relieved and angry. That my father was still able to function much of the time, that he was often charming and fun, very intelligent and sensitive, made our ambivalence a great source of guilt. I loved my father, and he loved us. His drinking was out of control, and so was our response to it.

What my sister, brother, and I learned were lessons often learned in an alcoholic home: don't ask for anything, don't talk about what's wrong, don't rock the boat, or, it's opposite, create a scene, (all or nothing). What many "adult children" learn is that we can count on no one but ourselves. We shrink from trusting, from "interdependence," from setting limits. We do not know our own limitations, we consider ourselves defective for being human. We identify with the underdog, thereby being wide open for manipulation by those who would take advantage of our often altruistic natures. Find a healer - nurse, doctor, therapist, social worker - and you will often find a person from an alcoholic home who has not developed problem-solving skills, let alone the art of negotiation.

I came to recovery because these beliefs and assumptions brought me pain. Worse, working as a nurse in a hospital fit quite nicely with those expectations: don't ask for what you need, don't talk about what's wrong. When I met the man who would usher me into "the program," as it is sometimes called, I said, "But I haven't lived with my father for 20 years!"

He, himself a recovering alcoholic replied, "You take it with you wherever you go. Alcoholism is a family disease."

Does that mean that it's not the drinker's responsibility, that the family is to "blame"? No. It means that we, having grown up under such circumstances, come to expect abuse as normal. We learn to accept unacceptable behavior as if we had no choice. We learn to see roller-coaster relationships (which bring out the adrenalin in us) as "happy."

The pain of such toxic living is bound to take it's toll, as it did for me. My need to control others, to be "hyper-vigilant" and watchful of their behavior to an extreme, to feel unappreciated, unwanted and alone - brought me pain. Through the kind and loving support of Alanon, Alanon-A.C.A. meetings, and with the help of therapy, I eventually learned new tools. I was able to take baby steps to change my behavior, and discovered how my patterns of living - the so-called "savior behavior" - were actually enabling poor situations to continue. Self-care, setting limits, insisting on being heard, were foreign concepts to me. Solution-seeking was not in my program - until I chose recovery.

Critics have said that such anonymous meetings are full of whiners who want to blame their parents, anyone, for their ills. It's true, some ventilation occurs and is good. However, the meetings focus on "experience, strength, and hope." These things mean taking stock, sorting out and acknowledging sources of strength, and offering hope from the good results of having tried new behaviors. Simply, it works.

Critics have said that the groups are against care-taking. This is not the case. However, as many caretakers, both professional and personal, see to the needs of others to the detriment of themselves - they become doormats. This is neither acceptable nor healthy. Such woeful patterns often end in great emotional and, often, physical pain. From that pain, we become desperate to try new ways.

The alcoholic who has landed in a destructive situation is often motivated by pain to attempt sobriety. As a "caretaker," I have had to learn that I must focus on my own life, on learning the genuine difference between nurturing and martyrdom. As a nurse, I have seen around me many people who did not know the difference. It is those to whom I write.

I also want to stress that although there is much suffering in my "family of origin," there was also much richness. My father was a great story-teller, and a nature-lover who was kind to others and wonderful to animals. We could take great, long walks together, hand in hand, discussing the world, the beauty of nature, the perfection of creation. From my mother, a physically beautiful and intelligent woman who had experienced many disappointments and tragedies, including having lived in an orphanage for a time while her mother - only fifteen years old - sought work, I learned my values. Values that included such things as not telling lies, being loyal to friends and loved ones, appreciating art, music and beauty. With the help of a Higher Power and life's generosity, and due to my own determination to grow, my relationship with her has improved in ways I never thought possible. Today, we know and respect each other's limits and we focus on our common ground of love.

My relationship with my father festered, broke open, and then before his death, finally metamorphised into truth and healing. He never admitted that his drinking had been a problem. But, he did admit to me, shortly before his last days, that he had "made a mess of things." I was able to be a participant in his dying process. I am grateful for that. In the end, the secrets were out, the truth was told, and the love remained.

The recovery efforts I have made are ongoing. There is no "cure." What are those new beliefs which help me to live a saner life?

I have learned I can:

* Respect others and be respected in return;
* Ask for help, for what I need. If I don't get it, it won't be the end of the world. What's more, it isn't because I am defective - God doesn't make junk!
* I can talk about what's wrong, seek relationships in which my needs are equally as important as others.
* I have the right to be heard, and I have a responsibility to be held accountable;
* I needn't accept unacceptable behavior;
* "No" is a complete sentence;
* Life is a process, a spiral rather than a straight line. People make choices. And, of course, we have "slips" - times in which we retreat to old and familiar behavior.

The hospital system is predicated upon nurses being obedient, silent, and submissive. We can discuss health care reform until we are "blue in the face," as my mother used to say, but without some change in the "family" structure, a move from authoritarianism to promoting resources and "empowerment," the true forces for healing will not be given room.

Hospitals need something and they need it fast: soul!

One nurse, Marlene Kramer, PhD, has done a study in which she sought the qualities of a facility which contributed to nurse retention. Nurses, it seems, universally wish that they were more appreciated, had greater autonomy, and more say in the health care arena.

Some hospitals studied seemed to satisfy nurses and stand in great repute. In these hospitals, nurses were salaried, had only one person to report to, and did not have to punch timecards. They took greater responsibility in terms of patient care, including clients ideas in their plans of care. Patient complaints decreased and nurse job satisfaction increased. At the same time, administrative perception of success expanded and costs were controlled. Nurses were seen as an equally important part of the team.

We don't want to be doctors. We don't want to give orders. Most nurses I know want to be creative, to be catalysts for health. We want to see a greater consideration for the MIND and SPIRIT of a patient, not just the body. We don't want to just "do to" someone, we want to "work with" someone, to engender his faith in his own healing process.

For years the JCAHO had on its panel physicians, dentists, pharmacists, and respiratory therapists. But this panel which determined the accreditation of, and set standards for hospitals and convalescent homes, had not a single Registered Nurse among its members. This changed in 1991!

Recovery and re-birth requires a kind of death. Death surrounded me, but I didn't start to understand its true value until ...

HER LAST BREATH - A WORD OF THANKS

She died and they all raised their arms and cried, great, loud, rolling cries. They danced the dance of grief, jumping up and down in unison, shaking their feet and flopping their heads. They fell on her and prayed. They said, "Oh, Mama, love you, Mama." They hugged her and caressed her forehead and said, "I'm sorry, Mama."

One of them, a nurse herself, came up to me and said, "We'd like to give Mama her bath; is there some place we can do it?

The holding room was empty. For how long, who knew? But at the moment, things were quiet.

We wheeled her back, covered in her white sheet - she was large and it took all four of us to do this - and I gave them basins and gowns and closed the door. The nurse daughter simply said thank you.

They were there for an hour. I looked in on them from time to time. This was a solemn washing, a bath of thanksgiving, the preparation of the body to cause a clean release of the spirit. The body could be released of all of its woes, here again loving strokes by daughters, daughters-in-law. Their singing was soft and yet strong, their prayers the prayers of thanksgiving. The face of the Mama was one of beauty and light; she had not suffered long; she was in a good place. When they left, the nurse-daughter clasped my hand and said again, "thank you. God bless you."

I was in awe of this process, which seemed so right, seemed so loving, and so spiritual. Acclaimed L.A. poet, Holly Prado has captured this idea in one of her poems, saying "death can't be a failure." (From, "Word Rituals" by Holly Prado, copyright, New Alliance Records, Los Angles, CA)

This is the way in which death used to be handled, not as a failure, but as part of life. As an event which put parentheses around that life, indulging it, making it a landmark in the lives of the remaining loved ones. Ten years later this experience was to serve as a guidepost for me at the moment of the death of one of my dearest friends. This is one of the most important and joyous memories of my nursing career. And to make it better, two days later we received a lovely card, thanking us for our kindness. It is proudly displayed, now yellow and a bit tattered, on my bulletin board. I will always be grateful that the nurse-daughter took the few moments to write the note.

Death death death death. The words sound like what it is - a simple but powerful fact of life.

And we are afraid. And we are all rowing our boats on top of it, we are all hearing it's echo, trying to create some music before we go ...

ONE NOTE

My bones
curve into a
rounded face, tree
of flesh.

My skin, soft,
pretending to be tough.
If you could see my gut it would quiver
with chattering
teeth.

If you could see my
heart it would curve
like upturned palm squeezing
juicy orange.

If I could see - I do see
what my blindness won't
reveal, the "how of it
of my true inner self,
my eyes would dart back and
forth like someone
hallucinating because of
one note, every note
possible, and possible
means nothing not even
probable
means anything. I am,
I must be made of actions, pulling
curtains, opening
letters, gritting teeth, slamming
doors, caught with
my pants down but squatting
with dignity.

HEALER

I love that dark bird
under your wizard's cape
as it flashes in wrath
and you lie in its wake,
in the dark rut of your
burned-out self,
the self that needs repair.

I am the healer
and
having healed,
am left alone
to lick my wounds.

I watch the road now,
recovering from the glare
wearing blinders against lost souls,
blinking to regain my vision.

Suzanne, RN 1985

A SUDDEN END

1991. George Bush was president. The idea of managed care and home health care was beginning to sprout from seed, and the California depression was being called an "economic slump." It was the year of the beating of Rodney King, the year that four police officers were arrested for his beating - two of whom I had worked with at another hospital. One of the officers was later judged guilty of the crime of depriving Mr. King of his civil rights. The other, in my opinion, should also have been called "guilty" - for he had worn a single black glove ...

The essay below was written in that year, just prior to my decision to take a personal leave from hospitals and from emergency nursing. I did so with a plan to move to another form of nursing. I tried working in an office, then in home health care and finally, in camp nursing.

The events which precipitated my decision to take leave have been documented here - being called a bitch for complaining about a physicians' tantrum; experiencing the continuing and mounting stress of legal, administrative, and staffing issues; being exhausted both professionally and personally.

If nurses could participate in the healing process at the bedside and be rewarded for hard work well-done, acknowledged by the hospitals in which they work; if hospital administrators included nurses in their planning and creating new avenues of delivering health care; if physicians became aware of the necessity of having experienced nurses on their team and refrained from behaving like spoiled children; and were not rewarded for doing so, this nurse might return. I realize that there are exceptions, but, during my years of service, such attitudes were the norm.

This book is about my path away from the bedside, which happened to coincide with my beginning recovery. The art of self-care was still a new concept for me, but meanwhile, the understanding that I needed a break was beginning to sink in. It is also about my strong advocacy for patients. But mostly, this is about my support of nurses, whose growth and empowerment, I believe will ultimately improve all other aspects of health care.

The message I had gotten over the years was loud and clear: "Don't speak about what's wrong." I had been suffering physical symptoms with increasing intensity: sleeplessness, early morning 4 a.m. panics which resulted in many of these notes. Symptoms had escalated from mere anxiety to crying spells before work, difficulty concentrating, and despair. I felt stuck, I felt sick, I felt tired.

Prayer, one of my biggest anchors, was even beginning to fail me. Before each shift, I sought a "healing attitude." Sometimes I would have to stop four or five times during a day to try to renew that perspective. It would not be the first time for such prayers. Nor would it be the last.

I WANT THE PEACE OF GOD

My gloved hands poured the alcohol. It doesn't kill the BAD germs, but I like the stringent fresh smell of it, the way the artificial grime lifts, the way it instantly dries, giving the semblance of cleanliness.

Here in emergency, cleaning helps not only to remove the stains of infirmity, it helps bring order from chaos. It is a ritual for nurses like myself who have tended to the inner and outer wounds of the souls whom chance directs here.

The linen and waste carts bear signs in Spanish and English, warning signs, protecting one against the danger of contamination.

Danger! Peligro! Contaminada!

I wipe them with the potion of cleanliness, seeing a new warning: our health care system is in trouble.

During fifteen years of nursing, I've cringed at the deterioration. The rules have changed and not for the better. The conditions of our patients seem worse. Emergency is being used as a clinic, a "holding" area, for sick patients who aren't sick enough to be admitted. Some H.M.O.'s regulate patients at the Emergency Room level, where most insurance companies continue to allow for the integrity of the ER doctors.

There is an increase in incidence of previously controlled communicable diseases, and children of all classes are not being properly vaccinated. In California, many patients treated in the emergency setting are immigrants, and a large portion of illegals come though the hospital doors in this and other border states. Poverty-related conditions - those which increase due to poor resources and poor knowledge - are all around us in this city of "angels."

Just as our culture manifests its own warning signs, addictions, homelessness, divorce, and apathy, so the medical system reflects this. We suffer from the results of bad habits and of the past (over indulging and under accounting) and are trying to come clean with a critical and often irresponsible public watching, indeed, seemingly hoping for mistakes. Now we have gone too far - and we are all in need. All of us, consumer and provider alike, are suffering.

Alanon and Alcoholic Anonymous teach recovery, not cure. They teach individual responsibility, moving from blame to choice and healthy action. In the same way that addictions and overindulgence and apathy are beaten - with honesty, limits, responsibility, incentive, and empathy - so must the repair of our health care system begin.

Let's look at some of the problems:

DOUBLE BLIND: Conscientious practitioners such as myself and the majority of those with whom I work, find ourselves in a dilemma. We are mandated to give excellent care, and, at the same time, insurance companies are reducing and/or limiting reimbursement. We must re-define "good" care. We see *some* health maintenance organizations providing the least comprehensive care possible, often combined with slipshod practices. This results in prolonged illness or return to hospitals due to premature release. It sometimes results in death when mismanaged by those who do not understand "quality." Good management forces us to be more prudent caretakers with quality as the goal. Bad management sacrifices optimum care. In fact, "optimum," in reality, exists only for the rich who can afford the "no-stone-unturned" approach.

THE TRIPLE BIND: A constant threat of lawsuit by the ever-vigilant legal system. Personal lawyers who advertise "Had a wreck" How's your neck?" capitalize upon the greed of irresponsible consumers who want a free lunch, and easy disability. This demeans the lawyers and the many conscientious practitioners who are competent and compassionate. We must stop this "scavenger" approach!

DWINDLING RESOURCES: Increasingly limited in their abilities to provide, to hire the proper members of ancillary personnel and nurses, to purchase needed equipment, hospitals are opting to refuse risk. Some are closing trauma centers or emergency services. Others are adding to the already dangerous nurse-patient loads, increasing risk of neglect or mistake. A nurse can competently care for a limited number of patients before she/he is forced to compromise standards. Hospitals are also dropping the kind of benefits from which hard-working nurses derive reward, and for which nurses are able to work with continued loyalty.

SATURATION: The elderly and the mentally ill have always suffered in our system. Now the workers and middle class clients are suffering as well. One despairing mother came to us because she had placed her son in a drug rehab center only to have him released early because his insurance ran out. I saw this happen at a psychiatric facility for which I had worked. I often wondered if harm was done with the disruption of care.

Standards have been unclear. It is time for all health "disciplines" to practice the art of healing, including a look into setting parameters which promote wellness from the outset. We all need to look at our practices with new eyes. Discharge planning, if integrated into each health care circumstance, will not only allow for the reduction of waste, but will also promote the appropriate use of all disciplines. Indeed, an optimal approach. In the meantime, many patients, relatives of you and me, find themselves in over burdened public systems, facing frazzled nurses and doctors who cannot do it all.

I mentioned earlier that some methods and attitudes which have helped people to overcome addictions can be used to begin setting right the ills of our system. I used to believe that if administrators were paid less and doctors drove less expensive cars, that all would be well. *This is far too simplistic.* As in family-centered recovery programs, the whole health care "family" must be treated.

What works?

First, we must **ADMIT DEFEAT**. The old ways are not working. *The present system is injurious to our health!*

Next, **EMPATHY**. Suspend blame and realize that most of us who give care and who receive it, have *good* intentions. Adversarial attitudes and threats estrange us from one another. It is time that consumer and provider learn to work together.

HONEST APPRAISAL. This system is not working! That other systems may be worse is not the point. Doctors and nurses feel unappreciated, patients feel endangered, and administrators feel confused. The problems won't go away by themselves. We must do an inventory of the facts. Look at ways to prevent the elderly and the mentally ill from having to fend for themselves alone. Look at ways in which the average American can afford to become well and stay well. This may mean that we all will have to take some responsibility for those less fortunate, but we are already doing so. A sliding scale system, or a percentage of income system might help. And, we must mandate that children will all have access to health care, no matter what!

APPROACH: IF WE EMBRACE A HEALING, SOLUTION-ORIENTED APPROACH, AS PATIENTS AND AS CAREGIVERS, WE BECOME PARTNERS-IN-HEALTH! This requires good communication, empathy and suspended judgment. I believe that each member of this society has a right to health care. However, *we must all do our part* to help to create a system which works. We cannot ignore any portion of our society in the planning.

INCENTIVE: Offer incentive to people to be well and stay well. Move the focus from "dis-ease" to "wellness." We are in an age when the mysteries of healing are being probed. Many answers point to the connections of body, mind and spirit. There is little doubt that one affects the other. Alternative practices such as acupuncture, hypnosis, biofeedback, and therapeutic touch must be re-examined by the medical community. These practices have seen wider use by the consumer. We have, in the past, relied too heavily on FDA approval. The fact of the matter is that certain treatments have proven themselves over time. The holdup is in the research costs and the ever increasing demand for research dollars. The competition has become fierce! This causes many worthwhile treatments to remain "unproven" by the scientific community.

A portion of the health care dollar must be allocated for research for less technological, but long-used, and known-to-be effective remedies. The art of healing does not require a space-age treatment, no matter how impressive. Let us remember that healing itself is still a mystery, and for centuries, has been an art. An integration of mind, spirit, and science is long overdue!

Other ways to improve health care must include expanded roles for nurses. So-called "extenders" to usual practice are on the rise. Home health nursing is one of the best examples of this type of approach.

RETURN TO WHOLENESS: We each have bio-psycho-social needs. I have often heard patients complain that they felt like a part instead of a whole. For the integration of the system, consider the following:

Participate with your providers and refuse to see nurses as handmaidens! "If caring were enough, anyone could be a nurse!" (an advertising slogan seen by the author in some nursing magazines). Our knowledge and judgment is paramount to the outcome of a patient's course!

Insist, through representatives and agencies, on being heard. Let lawmakers and policy makers know of your views! Think about what is missing, about what you wish would happen, and then think about your own solutions and state them!

Acknowledge that the years of education and discipline on the part of the physicians was sparked, most often, by the motivation to help people.

Empathize with administrators who must adhere to mountains of rigorous standards and requirements, titles and codes in order to bring you quality care.

Applaud the many technicians, social workers, pharmacists, housekeepers, and others, without whom hospitals could not exist!

Give constructive criticism. ATTACK THE SYSTEM, NOT THE PERSON. Learn good communication techniques.

Encourage help for impaired medical practitioners who need to address problems such as alcoholism or drug abuse. Give them firm limits and ways to become productive, while maintaining the safety of the consumer and co-workers.

Volunteer your services! Many hospitals are lacking in personnel to do the small things which make a difference.

Support. In the past, too many practitioner errors were ignored until the catastrophic event occurred. This set the tone for the legalistic approach we have today. We must move beyond the current out-dated system and into a more supportive setting. This new setting must hold those accountable who have violated the standards and patient rights, but it should find a supportive way to maintain a focus on critical patient care issues. Creative solutions to this or any crisis CANNOT begin in an atmosphere of fault-finding and belittling. Nor, does it help to keep your concern secret. Approach the person with compassion and with an eye towards solution regardless of whether the impairment be substance abuse or "burnout." Responsibility and self-esteem are the basis for all of these suggestions, for consumer and provider alike.

Finally, the subject of *Spirit* must be discussed. I'm not talking about religion, but rather considering the human heart which needs inspiration. Fellowships for drug and alcohol rehabilitation are based upon a belief that the higher good must prevail. Seek the greatest good in solutions. We all do this by taking responsibility, becoming the best we can be and encouraging others to do the same. Such accomplishment isn't easy, but it is simple.

I became a nurse for the human connection.

I became a nurse for the closeness, the touch.

I became a nurse for those moments when the edges of needing and giving are blurred by our human experience. We suffer, we *transcend, together*. It is the real drama of life, these intimate moments, which surpass fear, illness, or tragedy.

I became a nurse to help people. By doing so, I am not submerged in my own concerns. I see that some people have it better and some have it worse; that a dynamic exists and those who have it worse sometimes get better or pass through a state of Grace; those who have it better are no different from me, and human too.

I believe in love, discipline, and a higher good ...

The bin has been scrubbed well, and I prepare to end my day. It has been good to express these thoughts.

Someone else must feel the same. I don't know if it was a doctor, nurse or patient who wrote the words which startle me now. Words which I did not notice before, an incomplete sentence scribbled with wobbly letters beneath the stains, written anonymously, but very publicly. They say, simply:

I WANT THE PEACE OF GOD.

INSPIRATION

Soon after writing the previous essay, I was assigned to work a day in the Recovery Room. My restlessness was increasing, and the thought of leaving the bedside, perhaps forever, was troubling me. I wanted to leave my worries on the doorstep, and prayed for a healing attitude. I thought that I had achieved detachment, when I approached a lovely woman who was about to have surgery. She took me by the hand as she was being wheeled into the Operating Room and said, with a direct gaze and a rolling accent, "God bless you!" Something in me said a very heartfelt, thank you. Something in me was inspired to give my very best. The experience touched me deeply, and I wrote this poem.

SURVIVOR

God Bless You, she said,
reached for my hand,
gave me a kiss;
I am a survivor,
she said
from her sick bed.
my eyes turn away, tearful,
now looking,
they're her eyes, too.
God Bless You, she said,
I'm used to worrying,
be happy.

MESSENGER

I left the hospital - took a leave - hoping to find a new way. After first trying home health, then office nursing, them camp nursing (only boo-boos and bee stings), I took work as a waitress at a cappuccino bar (small, large, regular or decaffeinated, foam or milk, regular or non-fat, sugar or sweet-n-low?). On busy Saturday nights, I listened to great bands play. The most stress came from making foam! But, I needed better pay. This was the first year of a long-lasting economic slump in my state. Further more, I did not have a bachelors degree creating a bad position to be in when the competition is high.

During that time, I was forced to dip into retirement funds, at considerable penalty. The government would not allow loans against the funds. My financial situation continued to get worse. I had sent out numerous resumes to which no one responded. I applied to clinics where the policy was to hire L.V.N's for less pay. When I begged them to hire me, even at lower wages, they refused, citing policy. I heard that there were some research programs available, but the pay was a third of what I had been accustomed to making.

I came to realize that, while my choice to enter an A.A. degree program was useful in getting me out there as a single mother who must support her children, it did not serve me for the future. Still, when I look back on all the hectic days, raising them alone, working every other weekend and some nights, I realize that I had done all that I could do, and still had time to read stories at night and have a few moments to myself.

I became frightened that all doors upon which I had "knocked" seemed tightly closed. I panicked. I chose the inevitable.

There is an old Sufii proverb which questions all events, both "good" and "bad," by stating, after each - "who is to say whether this is a disaster or a blessing?" We do not always know the "big picture." Having faith and a recovery program or a religion or a philosophy, however, does not vaccinate us against suffering, or against pain.

I went back to the hospital.

Alanon teaches rigorous honesty in all of our affairs, unless it would deliberately hurt someone. What follows hurts me to tell it, but by doing so I might give substance to other nurses who experience a similar situation. First, let me say that throughout the years, I *had* built up a spiritual bank account. By that I mean that I had worked my fanny off - gone to meetings, read books on self-improvement, and spent time with positive, nurturing people, rather than pessimistic ones. Without these supports, what followed could have meant my demise.

Over the years, little by little, I had begun to shed the "savior behavior," the martyrdom I so often see in sister nurses. I took on a stronger, more effective way of living. However, having had my resources strained, I was once again with the same old "junk." I was faced with my habit of self-isolation and with the hospital's lack of resources for troubled nurses. It resulted in disaster.

The new hospital proved to be progressive, and busy. During my leave, however, nurses had taken on more responsibilities; drawing blood and blood gases were now added to the list of duties; cutbacks on the required number of lab personnel created these new responsibilities for the RN. The AIDS situation made it necessary to wear gloves to start IVs, something I'd previously done with ease. I could once start an IV on the first try just by feeling the vein, sometimes under layers of fat. The gloves proved ungainly and limited my sensitivity. I found myself tiring easily, experiencing an exacerbation of the immune-dysfunction syndrome.

I was rusty, my timing was off, and to further complicate the situation, personal tragedy took its toll. In the space of three months, two long-time friends passed away. Another with whom I had shared my introduction into the recovery offered by Alanon, acquired her second cancerous tumor. Only this time, it was bad. She had survived breast cancer, only to develop a totally new cancer in her pancreas. It was growing fast. I was loosing another of my best friends. The early morning panic attacks began anew, awakening me in a cold sweat. Crying spells, stomach pain, and irritable gut, my old friends, returned. "If I can only hold on." I told myself.

I was in denial about the truth of the matter. I was burned out, and needed to away from nursing entirely. I fought hard to stay on top of things. I fought to concentrate, to be the competent nurse I had once been. but, "the messenger doesn't stop until the message is delivered." I had trouble remembering orders, and once nearly gave the wrong patient medication. I neglected to place a strong medication on an electric pump - afterwards wondering why I had forgotten such a simple thing I fought to get hold of myself, but did not know where to turn.

Some co-workers asked if I needed help - but I wasn't sure what help to ask for. How does one ask for a return to former strengths? To have your gut stop churning? To have your best friend miraculously recover from impending death? To make the pain go away, to separate oneself from what the body is trying to say? That would have required entertaining the prospect of unemployment again - a truth which I fought.

I do not trust people easily and in this new place, there was no one with whom I believed I could share my fears. My co-workers were unable to confront me directly with their concerns. As a result, one morning, abruptly, I was given a list of my flaws which had accumulated over the course of my six-month stay. I was simply not cutting it. I had the terrible realization that I had been a subject of conversation. I, who had always been an asset, was now considered a hindrance. It cut to the quick. I felt impaled, the way one does by one's own humility.

It didn't matter that my physician, with whom I had worked years before in a very busy ER said, "Suzanne, I know you're a good nurse, I'd have you take care of me in a minute. You just need a break."

But I'd had a break. Then came the shattering of my self-image, of my identity. *If I were no longer a nurse, what was I?* With nowhere to turn, I called one of the social workers, who referred me to a crisis clinic.

When the counselor had me describe what I thought was going on, I blurted out, "I don't want to be there!"

Although I had drafted a list of solutions to my situation, and had not been asked to leave, in that moment it became clear, hospitals were no longer the place for me. I resigned my job, knowing that I was closing the door to receiving leave benefits.

This was life crisis. Not just burnout - but *loss*. At first, I thought that I would take a job at a doctor's office or clinic. But, each time the thought occurred to me, I would get chills and break out in a cold sweat. I was in the middle of a churning, wrenching despair which could no longer be ignored.

During my six weeks of crisis counseling, I pondered my decision and who I was, if not a nurse. I remolded my resume, trod the footpaths of the unemployed. I tallied my strengths. Retrieved memories of lost dreams. I drew more money out of my retirement savings, again, at considerable penalty. By now, the second Rodney King trial was underway, and we had a new president, whose wife was actually listening to nurses!

Before I had left the hospital, I had been asked by the medical director to research and develop a protocol for the recognition and treatment of victims of domestic violence. My last act as an employee was to present the results of those efforts. The presentation was well received. I had a tool to give to the community. and held tightly to it! With this task came a clearer picture of my inner landscape. I realized that the part about nursing which I enjoyed the most was providing patients with resources to help themselves.

My personal life was in a heartbreaking state. Not only had two friends passed away abruptly, but two others had moved away. My oldest son and I had suffered through an estrangement, and were newly reconciled. Now he was about to be married. My joy for him remains endless, but this was another passage with which to reckon. My younger son, living on his own, was working two jobs to be able to pay his rent. He had dreams of becoming an actor - and knowing what I know now about choices, about being true to oneself, I could never have discouraged him from that dream.

When I had returned to the emergency room, I had come across a quotation by an early Christian theologian, Meister Eckhart. The quotation affected me deeply and, it seems, prophetically. I had pasted it to the medicine cabinet beside a photograph of my two sons. It said:

> *"Treat all things as if they were loaned to you, without any ownership - whether body or soul, sense or strength, external goods or honors, house or hall ... everything."*

And indeed, it felt as if "everything" was leaving, falling away. My dear friend Carole, whose pain was increasing and her body was wasting minute-by-minute, was once again in the hospital for another treatment of her pancreatic cancer. Three weeks after leaving my job, after spending a busy morning distributing resumes, I went to the hospital where she had again been admitted.

In the car, exhausted, for a moment I thought, oh, maybe I'll wait for tomorrow. But a clear, strong voice within - the inner voice which I encourage all nurses to heed, said, "Go in there - NOW!" I am glad I did. As I arrived, Carole was dying. She was in a transition state, that fragile state between life and death, when one can hear but not respond. Her rapid breaths were labored, her eyes unfocused. I dropped my purse and briefcase, bent down and whispered close to her ear, "Carole, it's Suzanne. I love you."

Her breathing slowed and took on the irregular quality associated with impeding death. I turned to look at family members. They said nothing, but their eyes were anxious. Just then, she retched blood. Her mother left the room. I told her to call for the nurse on duty. I told her father, when her mother left, "she is going."

Five minutes after I arrived, Carole stopped breathing. The nurse came into the room and we nodded at one another. Carole had no pressure. A few cc's of bloody urine filled her foley bag. Her once shapely figure which had turned men's heads and sent them sighing - was now boney and frail. She shuddered, and another burst of blood came rushing from her mouth. I shall never forget the sight of my dear friend's lovely green eyes with such an empty stare, void of life, and seeing that dark trickle, oozing. I knew it was not longer our Carole, but what was left of her nearly 49 years. Like a shell she had finally shed, for no further work was to be done. She had been loaned to us, and now she was gone. Letting instinct again guide me, and remembering the experience in which I had seen a loving death in the emergency room, I gave her last rites. Then I called for a gown and a basin, and together, with another close friend, we bathed her. We removed the blood so that her mother would not have to remember it. We waited for the doctor to come in to make the formal pronouncement.

I did this all with an incredible calm. Carole had not attended Catholic services for many years, but during our last visits together, she had asked me to go to the chapel with her, where she had described the feeling of being "touched" by someone. Once, after such a trip to the chapel, we sat silently on bench just outside the doors. Carole turned to me and asked, "Did you just touch me?" I hadn't, but I know that something else had.

I had seen, surrounding her in those last days, a beautiful light, an incandescence, which signaled the presence of something greater than our bodies, our dreams. Despite her pain, there was a palpable sensation of "something more" which felt uplifting and grand. And Carole, felt it too, though we did not speak about it much, the effectiveness of words being lost to the understanding.

Only once before had I experienced such a moment.

I'd had to return to work as my father lay dying. I knew that he would be gone soon, but my time off was limited. Both my brother and I had gone to visit him and he had rallied, sat up, took off his oxygen, and smoked a final cigarette. Although he had summoned this energy, he could not walk nor rise from a semi-consciousness to say good-bye. I said to him, "Dad, I know it's selfish, but I am going to miss you."

He whispered in response, "Ah, Suzie, it's not selfish."

This marked one of only a few times in his life in which he had been able to be supportive. I weep as I write this, for the losses, for the gain.

That night, as I sat with a friend, I suddenly felt a strong sense of peace. The room grew brighter, and my friend, who saw it too, said, "Suzanne, something wonderful is happening." The feeling, like a great surge of love and beauty and illumination, lasted for a good thirty minutes. He and I sat in silence as it continued, and "touched" us, then slowly receded. I found out the next morning that my father had passed away at that moment. Even now as I write about these experiences, the remembrance is re-stimulated, the sensation of something ... *more.*

My tears for Carole did not come until later. But, when they came they came for her, for the friends who had preceded her in death and, also for a whole time frame of my life which was now falling away before my astonished eyes.

In the previous year my relationship with a man with whom I had spent five years, the man who had been with me when my father died, ended. At the end of our relationship, during a fight and brief absence from one another, his father had died suddenly. He said that he decided not to tell me, but circumstances brought him to my door. As he came to the end of the street on which I lived, the chain on his motorcycle snapped. He ended up pushing it the block to my apartment. Thus, the deaths of our fathers had marked the beginning, and the end, for us.

Life was making a strong statement now, which I could no longer ignore. Time to change, time to die a little, and be ushered into a new phase of life, with time to add to the story. The late psychoanalyst, Carl Jung, has said that neurosis is caused by the "interruption of a person's story." (From ***Jung And The Story Of Our Time***, by Laurens Van Der Post). These sudden endings have made me look at my own. Recurring events, dreams, words, threads, create a pattern. Once upon a time, there was a small bright girl who was sensitive and artistic and lonely. She took on some burdens which were heavy for a child - and in later life she needed to learn to let go. Even if the burdens felt like friends ...

I look back and try to retrieve what was lost. Try to keep what is good and continue to write ...

Something in me is, and will always be, a nurse. *Thank God there is more than one way to serve!*

THE NEW NURSING FEMINISM

Despite my disappointments and "failures," I feel empowered. One day I may return to those infirmary halls, but now is the time to look at a new idea which has emerged, a pattern for my life, and perhaps yours. The idea is of a "new" feminism.

Gloria Steinem, world-famous feminist, wrote most recently that true self-esteem must come from personal insights, true power from self-esteem, "like a spider spinning her web, we create much of the outer world from within ourselves." (***Revolution form Within, A Book of Self-Esteem***, p.8).

Nursing empowerment begins with personal empowerment. How does one attain it? What are the characteristics? What are the limitations of personal empowerment?

As it turns out, the "solution" lists which I wrote more than two years ago remain accurate today. A few things have changed. Nurses have become more aware of their increased ability to be a stronger voice. And so it should be. But some other behaviors must lead to empowerment if nurses are to be heard.

The physician who had a tantrum and shoved the tube down the drunk patient's nose was suffering from burnout. He did apologize to me before I left. He, too, found himself in a different career.

Physicians at the last hospital where I worked had a no-abuse policy. If any doctor was abusive to a nurse, her or she would be called on it. Amazing! I saw nurses more regularly as team members, and witnessed the growing trend towards managed care, but with a difference. Nurses such as myself with years of experience, are using their knowledge to see to it that, in addition to being cost-effective, care is also timely and appropriate. Nurses are also acting in more autonomous ways in the roles of practitioners, nurse anesthetists, while more hospitals are downsizing, and cutting costs. Nurses are moving to the outpatient theater - where physicians deigh to go.

Recently proposed California legislation would require physicians to have instruction on topics such as human sexuality, acupuncture, nutrition, and domestic violence. Many physicians have not received exposure to these topics in medical school, residency, or fellowships. This would be an improvement, long-called for by nursing. Patients can only benefit from such policies.

Nurses have far to go. As long as physicians, male or female, believe that they can yell at a nurse, throw an instrument, ignore a nurse's input, as long as patients who are able still say "wipe me," as long as administrators can fire a nurse for protesting about an abusive family, as long as the media ignores the very important contribution of nurses now and over the years, then we have big work to do. And, it all begins with self-empowerment.

So, what is Nursing Feminism? It is the result of acknowledging that nurses are the most numerous participants in medicine whose collective voice is inherently strong. It is the result of nurses BECOMING AWARE of what is unacceptable behavior and refusing to participate in situations which will be detrimental to the nursing cause as patient advocates. Nurses must be an EQUAL professional team member.

Certain nursing situations such as "floating" to unfamiliar departments and working double shifts on required overtime are dangerous to clients and the nurse. Worse, these practices put the nurse in the position of "scapegoat." If anything goes wrong, her license is on the line. If she refuses, her job is on the line. A nurse cannot win in these kinds of circumstances.

Before nurses can handle such a situation, we must be familiar with the concept of self-care. A nurse who values her job and her license will take a stand. However, she must know first that she is allowed to be an adult and make such a choice for the patients. Nurses are full of guilt and often react to outrageous requests as a child would react to a parent. It takes a lot of courage to say to a physician who orders a medication which you know is not cleared to be given intravenously, that you are uncomfortable giving it. Many times before I had seen the drug Demerol given intravenously, I had to take a stand and hand it to the doctor to give. When I knew that it could be given and in what doses, I became comfortable, but not at first. Confrontation was usually uncomfortable, but for a person with little self-esteem, it can be a disaster.

Personal strength grows in situations where we make the commitment to stand in our advocacy, in our caution, if need be. The way we sabotage our position is by treating each other badly. Time and time again, we hear, at the change of shift, derision and criticism. "Why wasn't this done? You guys always leave a mess!" Or we hear gossip. Or we see triangle situations: J. talks about L. behind her back, but they are nice to each other face to face. And, while we are bickering, administration continues to limit autonomy, refuse pay raises, adds patients to the short-staffed floors, and take away benefits.

If nurses want, *really want*, to have a voice, then we must earn to deal with conflict, stand together on issues such as short-staffing and floating, benefit reduction and so on. It takes energy to come to terms with nursing issues. The ultimate benefit is a strong voice, visibility. Nursing supervisors must begin to support the integrity of nurses while guiding them to solutions, rather than automatically adopting the "management" point of view. Nurses are capable of much more than being treated like recalcitrant children.

At the root of nursing impulse is the creative sensibility and sensitivity which brings us to the "calling" of the profession in the first place. Give nurses a place in policy-making and ethics discussion meetings. Give us a place to do what we do best - finding ways to help patients to help themselves. Provide a supportive atmosphere for nurses, and we will give our very best.

Nursing empowerment begins with ourselves. Below are some alternatives to futile behavior. Behavior which limits and dis-empowers nurses. Consider the following definition:

POWER: (n)

1. The ability to do something;
2. vigor, energy, strength;
3. a property, great *healing* power;
4. control, influence.

In its definitions of power, nowhere does the ***Oxford American Dictionary*** mention the word aggression, nor does it mention the words martyrdom or sacrifice.

Most nurses are well-meaning and caring. The aggressors of the world have less empathy, we can fill our pockets with it! We are also smart, efficient. But, despite all of our achievement, our intelligence, our compassion, we (many of us) suspect, deep down inside, that we are really not good enough, smart enough, or clever enough to be treated well. We know that something is wrong, but we continue to do things the way we had always done them, hoping that, somehow, it will all get better.

The cure, which is within us, requires small deliberate steps. The reward is in effectiveness, being heard. Instead of sacrificing, backstabbing, taking abuse, using covert games and power trips, stuffing our feelings with food, alcohol, tobacco or drugs, not taking care of ourselves, overreacting or underreacting - we can choose the following:

1. Make self-care our first priority. (Norwood, paraphrased).
2. Recognize that anger and fear are inner guides which signal that a personal boundary may be being violated. (Goldhor).
3. Recognize that angry "blowup" is not usually effective except to ventilate our tension. (Goldhor).
4. We can use our feelings to tune in to what we need - and make a request based on that. (Goldhor).
5. We can be heard by speaking up respectfully and ask for what we want and see what we get. (Alanon).
6. We can be determined not to treat others disrespectfully; in doing so we loose our credibility.
7. We can choose not to participate in destructive or liable behavior. Gandi said, "non cooperation is directed not against men, but against measures. ("Principles, not Personalities," A.A.).

8. We can take care of ourselves by taking breaks when we need them, getting enough sleep and exercise. (In eight years at one hospital, rarely did I get a full half-hour lunch break.).
9. We can be honest, *privately* with co-workers when we feel the FIRST moment of friction.
10. We can choose not to accept unacceptable behavior.
11. Using "I" messages is one way to make strong, clear statements. "I need you to help me when you have a minute." "I am not able to help you right now but I'll be there when I'm done here." (Gordon).
12. Mean what we say and say what we mean.
13. Accept that we are human; deal with our mistakes promptly, find ways to prevent their recurrence without sinking into self-pity. When confronted with my difficulty in the ER, I thought about the best way for everyone to win. I could have stayed, made some goals for myself, but, after self examination, I chose to resign. Still, choices needn't always be so dramatic.
14. Stop beating ourselves up. This takes work!
15. *Trust your gut*; nurses were born with a sixth sense - we can make it work for ourselves.
16. Arrive on time, leave on time, contribute to the team effort, follow the path of healthy self-discipline. "Without discipline we can solve nothing." (Peck).
17. Acknowledge the good of others.
18. Questions are a good way of clarifying conflicts. "What assignment would be fair with you?" "Do you have a problem with the way I'm doing things?" "Is there something that you want from me?"
19. We can try not to take everything so seriously. "Choose your battles!"
20. Ask, "How important is it?" State, "First things first." (Alanon).
21. Attend twelve-step meetings if alcoholism or compulsive behavior play an uncomfortable role in our lives.
22. Stop "overfunctioning" (Goldhor) and taking responsibility that belongs to others. This is hard at first, then it can be fun.
23. Avoid ultimatums, often premature and ineffective, and learn about assertiveness, negotiation. Read, take courses, then begin small steps toward progress.
24. Support each other!

Recovery from martyrdom and helplessness has some payoffs and it has a price. The price is that we have to give up some behavior which made our "role" easier. Speaking up for our own needs and setting limits means that we don't get to feel like victims. A feeling that some of us are very familiar with.

As we practice these behaviors, as we learn to speak up, the ability becomes catching, the greater our self-esteem. We learn to seek solutions, we become effective, and we are heard!

Begin with an affirmation: *I trust in the process of life. I am respectable and respectful. I am effective. I am powerful. I am caring. I am a nurse.*

Chapter Resources

1. Lerner, Harriet Goldhor, (1985),***The Dance of Anger***, Harper & Row
2. Lerner, Harriet Goldhor, (1989),***The Dance of Intimacy***, Harper & Row
3. Beattie, Melody, (1989), ***Beyond Codependency***, Harper-Hazeldon
4. Seabury, David, (1937), ***The Art of Selfishness***, Simon & Schuester
5. Norwood, Robin, (1985), ***Women Who Love Too Much***,
6. LeMon, Cal, (date unknown), ***Assertiveness: Get What You Want Without Being Pushy***, National Press Publications
7. ***The Oxford American Dictionary*** (1990)
8. Peck, Scott, (1978), ***The Road Less Traveled***, Simon & Schuster
9. Shalla, Shalu, (1991), ***Quotes of Gandi***, All India Press
10. The literature and meetings of Alanon Family Groups
11. ***The Big Book of Alcoholics Anonymous***
12. Overeaters Anonymous
13. De Angelis, Barbara, (1992), ***Revolution from Within - A Book of Self-Esteem***, Little, Brown

MORE THOUGHTS ON REFORM

Questions:

1. Are we willing to change "the system"?
2. What are we willing to change for the greatest good?
3. Is our technology making it difficult to keep the "heart" in health care? If so, how do we replace it?
4. Do we think that a legal approach to dying will make it any easier to experience?
5. Is there some way, besides the mind-set of dollars and cents, in which we can find answers?

These questions came to me in pondering the changes which have been proposed by the multitudes of interest groups who would have their considerations be given a voice. It is time, in our great "reformation", to reject practices which do not honor our integrity, our right to choose, and our humanity. If we are seeking solutions, we must not loose sight of those fundamental elements. We need to educate ourselves about humane treatments, as opposed to "glamorous" ones. Patients need to be acknowledged, their situations recognized. Pain control, spiritual needs, family needs cannot be neglected in the provision of "treatment". We must ask ourselves how we want to die - and whether we want to experience our last moments, if indeed a choice is given, tangled in wires and tubes, or be allowed to die peacefully in a less technological setting. We must decide if insurance companies or the government must pay for experimental treatments, merely to try to prolong life, with the thought that a "miracle" might happen, or whether it is better to allow a terminal disease process to follow a "natural" course.

We must think about where our research dollars are going, and about the morality of experiments with animals, fetuses, or genes. We must realize that the high cost of drugs makes it practically impossible for the poor and elderly to pay for them, and whether drug companies should create a fund for such social considerations.

We must decide how to create humane methods of reimbursement. If review and management are the answer - and this appears to be the case, whether through government-run programs or insurance policies - how should they be run? Do we choose "products" like we choose a car, or do we allow for a myriad of choices? Do we pay for those who are below a certain income level, or continue to let them "fall through the cracks'? Must small businesses be as responsible as big ones in the overall plan to develop a congruent solution? What are we as Americans willing to accept? Waiting for services? Rationing of services? Conservative treatments? Prudence in treatment has been deemed by some as miserliness, or worse, neglect. Withholding of treatments has been deemed to be cause for "damages" - and lawyers reap the rewards. Just because we have a technology, is it wise to use it? Is it adding to the art of healing, or suppressing it?

Does the suppression of one care-giving group for the interest of another promote benefits to patients, or reduce them? We are all potential "consumers"; in restoring the "soul" to health care, these very important questions must be asked. No one is let off the hook, here.

One thought continues to return to me. Until we are able to recognize the great mystery of life, which includes death, we will not find "solutions". Our constant return to "economics" and "science", without the balancing considerations of philosophy, spirit, and soul, will constantly hinder the process.

The bigger picture must be considered. It is my belief that if we begin to honor nurses as "healers", whose instincts exemplify something sacred in society, indeed, in the world, then answers will start to come. Treat us as a most treasured resource, and we will find creative ways in which to participate fully in this great mystery. See nurses as alchemists whose offering includes but also transcends pure "science", and enters the realm of art, poetry, and beauty. See this, reward this, honor this. In England, nurses in uniform are able to ride free on public transportation. Instead of "National Nurse's Week" we could have a "Nightingale Celebration" all year round. Hospitals would nurture their precious resources by offering support, good parking spaces, nurses advocacy programs, free medical care for nurses. Businesses could offer nurse discounts, scholarships, trips. All in honor of those who have served with intelligence, efficiency, creativity, and most of all, with the greatest impulse of human nature - to ease the suffering of others.

"Assembly of Japanese Bicycle Require Great Peace of Mind."
Robert Pirsig, ***Zen and the Art of Motorcycle Maintenance***, Bantam New Age Books.

THE ZEN OF NURSING

Peace of mind eludes us. At the end of a day, of a week, a month, a year, what is your feeling about your job? Are you usually serene, satisfied? Or are you left with lingering physical and emotional pain? Nurses who work hard, feel unrewarded in the light of the hospital "system". One nurse to I whom spoke discussed how guilty she felt for taking a day for herself instead of helping her sister with a problem. A single day! This was an extremely competent nurse who not only worked hard but spent one of her days off volunteering for a charity. Her family expected her to be the care-taker, no matter what other responsibilities she had. She was the rock of whatever - and no one else in the family shared the task. The situation, constantly serving other's needs at the expense of her own, was causing her pain. She was suffering from ill-placed guilt. She was the oldest in the family, an added "role" achieved through no fault of her own. But, now it was taking its toll. Dark circles grooved beneath her eyes; she was tired! Serenity was a fleeting feeling at best.

Another nurse I knew who was *Miz One Nurse Show,* loved the challenge of taking on a big load. The more trauma the better. She was quick, efficient, loath to tolerate self-care in others. Just pile on the work, I can handle it by myself! was her motto. One night, through no fault of her own, a patient fell out of bed. She had been working alone, and was tending a heart patient when the incident happened. The railing, which had needed repair, just gave way - and Kaboom! The patient did not suffer any injury, not even a bruise, but the nurse was a basket case when she told the story to us the next morning. You'd have thought she had killed someone. But her tears were real.

Serenity is a personal thing. Nurses often suffer needlessly from too high expectations, too little understanding of what self-care means.

In ***Zen and the Art of Motorcycle Maintenance***, the character asks, "And what is good, Phaedrus, and what is not good? - need we ask anyone to tell these things?"

Part of serenity is being here and now. Part of finding serenity is recognizing the truth, for ourselves, of a situation, place, or thing. Understanding the truth - not denying it - of the darkest thing, helps us to know what to do about it. Does the positive outweigh the negative? We might choose to stay. Does the voice, "I don't want to!" come in, despite our wishes to make something good or acceptable? Then we must listen, and then make our choices. A ride on a motorcycle can be fun, also dangerous. The ride can possibly be interrupted by mechanical problems, possibly too cold, possibly full of a feeling of freedom. Serenity comes from paying attention to what is true for us. This takes commitment to ourselves, it takes patience with ourselves. Buddhists call such paying attention "mindfulness," and many believe that serenity and even "enlightenment" can be the result.

Once I attended a Sting concert. It was in a crowded auditorium and I could barely see him due to the angle at which I was sitting. And I usually don't like big, crowded places. But I found myself so involved with it that an insight into the very meaning of life happened as I listened to his music. Afterward I told my friend, "You might think that this is silly, but while I was listening, I had the feeling that nothing - no problem in this life - mattered." My friend turned to me, incredulous. "I had the same feeling!" he said. Being mindful of the music had created an unexpected illumination.

There are many ways to practice "mindfulness." Buddhist practices are many and varied. Examples include espousing a form of meditation called *zazen*, or chanting *daimoku*, singing "*Nam myo ho, ren ge kyo*" and asking for wisdom. Other western ways of attaining mindfulness are also a path to knowing one's inner truth. A nurse with whom I worked served in Vietnam. She described her many beautiful antiques to me. They had been passed down from generation to generation. She obviously relished them. But, then she told me, "We have a saying, which we used in Vietnam. 'It don't mean nuthin.'" If she had to part with her furniture, she felt she could do it. "I have things in perspective," she said. "Life is what counts."

Others turn to prayer, to dance, to study. *Serenity is perspective.* It is accepting what is, at a given moment, and not trying to make it something else. Serenity does not mean being immune to the suffering of life. It does not mean being above it all. *It is about staying with the self, and the highest good, one day at a time.* The Zen of nursing would mean staying with your responses to the daily work, and learning to be mindful of what they might mean.

My last shift was in a busy downtown Los Angeles Emergency room. I had a room with five monitored beds. Suddenly, five paramedic runs came in, back to back. We were deluged with patients, including two fresh traumas. Patients were doubled in the hallways. All of my patients were on monitors; I was tending a very dehydrated sick child. All of the nurses were as busy as I looked up across the hallway and saw one of the two physicians looking out over the mess. His face had a look of shock. "Where do I start?" he seemed to be saying. The look on his face reflected my own bewilderment. All I could do was to prioritize. I had a sick child in front of me. I started an IV, drew labs. Between tasks, scanned the monitors of the other patients hoping, praying no one would get a dysrhythmia.

No one did. The next shift arrived, just in the nick of time ... but I will never forget the look on the doctor's face. Working at the bedside often IS that look. It IS that up-to-our-knees-in-alligators feeling. It is also a sigh when it is all done, when the quiet returns. But *my* response to that cycle had changed. The look on that doctor's face solidified what I knew. It was over. I am done. Now, when I hear a siren, I cringe. Me, as an organism, reacts as if to noxious stimuli. Me, as a being, doesn't want the responsibility, the chaos, the "excitement", any more.

Robert M. Pirsig writes in ***Zen and the Art of Motorcycle Maintenance***, that "Buddha, the Godhead, resides quite as comfortably in the circuits of a digital computer or the gears o a cycle transmission as he does on the top of a mountain or in the petals of a flower. To think otherwise is to demean the Buddha - which is to demean oneself." If we pay attention to the small sources of awareness, and thus pave the way for self-care, we will become able to reach for tools to use or know when it is time to move in another direction. We will also be able, more fully, to appreciate the fine moments of any activity.

One such moment came as a student nurse. Taking care of my first patient, who was in end-stage kidney dysfunction, I was frustrated about my inability to get the tasks done on time. But a friendly veteran nurse came in and helped. Suddenly I was loving the sound of sheets being smoothed and folded, loving the neat, crisp appearances of them, reflecting light against the dull walls, loving the rhythm of healing. I was loving the sigh of the patient as he put his head on the soft pillows and fell almost immediately asleep. Small but beautiful moments, which kept me at the bedside for a long time. They were moments of light.

My body doesn't want to do it right now, but when I think of nursing, I can still find serenity in those memories. One day, I may go back, or work in a voluntary capacity, but it will be a while. Me, in relation to it, just doesn't fit right now. And that's the "Zen" for me.

None of us needs answers, really. Sometimes we just need new ways of looking at things. Or a voice to remind us of what we already know. Zen, or serenity, is not about avoiding pain. It is about finding out what that pain means. Or, if it outweighs the joy. Or, if it means "nuthin."

What is the sound of the art of nursing? Or, in a form of vernacular, "What's it for you?" And be it, one day at a time.

No matter what form it takes, I am a nurse. And I like the sound of that.

GHOST

I have fed the hollow dry mouths.
I have bathed the corroded
crevices of the unloved,
the unwanted.

I have genuflected
as addicts stare wall-eyed,
seeing one, two, three
of me, before
snorting awake, calling me bitch, hating
the hands which rouse them from death.

I have washed the feet of transients,
dented with stones, covered with maps.
I have bailed the pools of
scarlet tidal waves,
poured from beneath jaundiced eyes.
"so this is it," they say, between
bloody retchings. "I bleed, you tend me.
"I think I am dying."
and then, "Who tends to you?"

I wring out the cloth of a thousand missions
and hang it out to dry,
a faded dream.
I put it into the closet, with the bloodied, scuffed shoes,
I bite into an apple, and see the millions;
I hold a grain of sand, and hear them cry;
the ghost of me is in those rooms,
it was she who did it, who nursed the sick -
not I, no longer, I.

Suzanne, RN

To honor the life-saving help she received as a grateful member of Alanon, Suzanne has chosen to publish this book anonymously.

THE TWELVE STEPS

1. We admitted we were powerless over alcohol - that our lives had become unmanageable.
2. Came to believe that a Power greater than ourselves could restore us to sanity.
3. Made a decision to turn our will and our lives over to the care of God *as we understood Him.*
4. Made a searching and fearless moral inventory of ourselves.
5. Admitted to God, to ourselves and to another human being the exact nature of our wrongs.
6. Were entirely ready to have God remove all these defects of character.
7. Humbly asked Him to remove our shortcomings.
8. Made a list of all persons we had harmed, and became willing to make amends to them all.
9. Made direct amends to such people wherever possible, except when to do so would injure them or others.
10. Continued to take personal inventory and when we were wrong promptly admitted it.
11. Sought through prayer and meditation to improve our conscious contact with God *as we understand Him*, praying only for knowledge of His will for us and the power to carry that out.
12. Having had a spiritual awakening as the result of these Steps, we tried to carry the message to others, and to practice these principles in all our affairs.

SUGGESTED READING LIST

SELF HELP:

1. Lerner, Harriet Goldhor: (1985), ***The Dance of Anger***, Harper and Row.
2. Lerner, Harriet Goldhor: (1989), ***The Dance of Intimacy***, Harper and Row.
3. Beattie, Melody: (1989), ***Beyond Codependency***, Harper Hazelden.
4. Seabury, David: (1934), ***The Art of Selfishness***, Simon & Shuster.
5. Norwood, Robin: (1985), ***Women Who Love Too Much***
6. Peck, Scott: (1978), ***The Road Less Traveled***, Simon & Shuster.
7. Steinem, Gloria: (1992), ***Revolution From Within - A Book of Self-Esteem***, Little, Brown.
8. Gordon, Thomas: (1970, 1075), ***Parent Effectiveness Training***, Signet Plume.
9. ***The Big Book of Alcoholics Anonymous***
10. ***The Slogans of AA, and Alanon Family Groups***, public domain.*

INSPIRATIONAL:

11. Iyer, Raghavan (editor): (1993), ***The Gospel According to Thomas***, Concord Grove Press.
12. Van Der Post, Laurens: (1975), ***Jung and the Story of Our Time***, Vantage Books.
13. Persig, Robert: (1974), ***Zen and the Art of Motorcycle Maintenance***, Bantam New Age Books.
14. Dillard, Annie: (1977), ***Holy the Firm***, Harper Colophon Books.
15. Fox, Emmett: (1934, 1966), ***The Sermon on the Mount - The Key to Success in Life***, Harper, San Francisco.
16. Shalla, Shalu: (1991), ***Quotes of Gandhi***, All India Press.
17. de Saint Exupery, Antoine: (1943, 1971), ***The Little Prince***, Harcourt Brace Jovanovich.
18. Fremantle, Francesca & Chogyam Trungpa (translation): (1987), ***The Tibetan Book of the Dead - The Great Liberation Through Hearing in the Bardo***, Shambala Publications, Inc.
19. Borges, Jorge Luis: (1962), ***Labyrinths***, New Directions Publishing Corporation.
20. Waters, Frank: (1963), ***Book of the Hopi***, Penguin Books

TAPES:

21. Prado, Holly (1972), "Larger Than Other Plants," From: "Word Rituals," 1993 New Alliance Records, Lawndale, California.

* Twelve-step programs have no authority at the level of press, radio, or television. "Out public relations policy is based on attraction, rather than promotion; we need always to maintain personal anonymity at the level of the press, radio, TV, and films. We need guard with special care the anonymity of all AA members." The 11th tradition of Alcoholics Anonymous.

This author presents only her experience, strength, and hope. Take what you like and leave the rest.

A CARETAKER'S JOURNAL

♥ ♥ ♥ ♥ ♥

Dear Colleague,

A journal is a wonderful place to write your thoughts, feelings, experiences, pain, frustrations ... even a poem that describes how you feel. My journal has been a place for me to keep my thoughts and feelings together for many years and through this book, bring them to you. My hope is that they will help many nurses who have faced the guilt and pain of deciding to leave the profession that we love.

It is my way of saying "it's OK." My way of saying there is a way to recover and to move on with your life.

I hope that your words will one day help other nurses. Use these journal pages to begin your own healing process.

Sincerely,

Suzanne

A CARETAKER'S JOURNAL

A CARETAKER'S JOURNAL

A CARETAKER'S JOURNAL

A CARETAKER'S JOURNAL

A CARETAKER'S JOURNAL